Riding the Rainbow Through the Storms

A Colorful, Humorous Story of Recovery

Mrs. Viola B. Collins
and
Janice Marie Collins, Ph.D.

Riding the Rainbow Through the Storms
A Colorful, Humorous Story of Recovery
Chicago, Illinois
Copyright 2023 Janice Marie Collins
ISBN 978-0578935-37-9
ISBN 978-0578935-36-2 (epub)

Table of Contents

1   Living and Writing in Our Purpose............................ 5
2   My Mother 7
3   The Day Things Changed...................................... 14
4   It's a Long Way to Z 19
5   NOOOOOOOOO...ZZZZZZEEEEEYYYYYYY 25
6   A Shopping We Will Go 27
7   The Freedom Rides 31
8   It's the Small Things 36
9   Stories from El Cuatro de Bano 39
10   The Buddy System 42
11   OOOOPPPPPPSSSSSSS 44
12   It is *too* Raining.. 49
13   Losing Track of Time 53
14   The Real You: When It Comes Blurting Out........... 55
15   Your Biggest Fan: Manipulation Begs Attention 58
16   It's Not Easy Being Me 60
17   The Biting Effect 62
18   And Another Thing.. 64
19   Use It or Lose It.. 69
20   It's All in the Head 71
21   Everyone Do-si-do! 76
22   Keep Moving 78
23   Things to Remember.. 80
24   Don't Miss It... 84
25   And Don't Forget... 86
26   Dignity 91
Bonus   My Daddy, Mommy's Baby: Lessons from My Father........... 96
     Lessons From Our Father Who Art In Heaven 104
     The Spirituality of It ALL 104
     About the Author.. 115

Living and Writing in Our Purpose

So many survivors as well as their caregivers feel all alone when going through something as traumatic as a stroke. My mother and I noticed the need for a tool that offered some safe advice and good old hope to others in similar circumstances. With that in mind, we decided to write this book. Before my mother passed in 2002—possibly picking up an infection during a hospital visit—I'd ask her questions like, "Mommy, if you could tell people what it takes to make it through, what would you tell them?"

I wrote her responses down, along with what I learned from caring for her and how others worked their magic. This process began the first notes for this book.

As a family, we created a magic carpet that took us on a colorful rainbow ride through this storm. Everything that was taken away from Mommy, we worked to find it again; and it ALL came back. She may have walked a little differently, danced a little differently, even spoken a little differently through word selections tied to an unfiltered emotional base, but she came back! Although it wasn't easy, I can honestly say, at the end of it all, it was absolutely worth the effort. Now, we share our story with you.

Although my mother passed while we were just beginning to write this book, it was important that I followed through. The lessons we learned are still pertinent and can be helpful for others. I think of Mommy at least once a day. I laugh, smile and have conversations with her in my head about how great of a ride we had. If she were here today, I know she would feel the same, laughing at what we went through and came through.

We pray and hope that as you read our story, you are encouraged to laugh as well and create your own magic carpet ride of triumph the best way you can. If you happen to learn something from our experiences, our prayers have been answered. Just remember, you can make it through and, as my mother used to always say, when things get tough, "Keep moving. Don't let the grass grow under your feet and, when you are feeling down, no matter what, keep looking up!"

I encourage you to ride the rainbow that sits behind the storm. Whether or not a pot of gold is waiting for you is not the focus. Stay present. A colorful ride is just around the corner. May God bless you and always keep you near.

CHAPTER 1

My Mother

My mother, Mrs. Viola B. Collins grew up addressing challenges at a very young age. Her parents, Addie B. Watson and Clarence Burrell divorced when she was in pre-school. Until the age of twenty-two, my mother lived with her father Clarence Burrell and his mother—her grandmother—Addie Ewell. Her father was an influential citizen and respected man of God in his Churchill neighborhood. Although both of my mother's parents lived in Richmond, Virginia neighborhoods close in proximity (her mother lived in Maymont), Mommy spent very little time with her mother.

Mommy was brought up in a strict and religious household. She was always well dressed, fed and well-mannered. Her high-quality surroundings included Victorian furniture and antiques passed down through the family in pristine condition. In her father's home, she was not allowed to date, wear pants or to miss church services; the decorum in the household was very proper. She had to be ladylike without exception.

My great-grandmother (her father's mother), who passed away around the age of 106, was very ladylike as well, with a nice smile and beautiful skin. My mother's father was always well dressed in nice slacks, polished shoes, an ironed shirt, bowtie and perfectly groomed hair. He strolled each day for exercise and smoked one pipe in the evening. That is how I fell in love with the smell of tobacco rising smoothly from a beautifully made pipe.

Throughout my entire life, although my mother called her father "Daddy," I never heard my grandfather call my mother anything but Mrs. Collins. Mommy was his only child. It was a strict household, yet his love was felt in other ways, and Mommy made sure we visited him on each trip we took to Richmond. Because of the divorce, we—the children—didn't learn a great deal about his side of the family, but the relatives we met were kind, nice, funny, well-dressed and well-mannered, of course.

As soon as Mommy turned twenty-two, she moved in with her mother and her stepfather, John Jasper, who we lovingly called Big Mama and Big John. Mommy was extra special in the Watson family, because she was the first grandchild. She received a lot of physical love and affection from her mother and Big John and her nine-year-old half-sister, Jacqueline—our aunt Jackey. This will be the only time I will use the word "half" when speaking of Aunt Jackey, because there wasn't and isn't anything "half" about any part of her. Her love, affection, support, guidance and hugs were always full for my mother, my daddy and all my brothers and sister. Always and forever.

When visiting her mother, Mommy also received a lot of love and affection from her cousins, aunts, uncles and family members who were always getting together for updates, good food, dancing and laughs.

Mommy was always independent. While working full-time at Virginia Mutual Insurance Company, she put herself through the Smith-Madden Business College in Richmond and earned a degree in Secretarial Science. Highly intelligent, she took classes in shorthand, accounting, business law, speed reading, business management, business machines, salesmanship, English, typing and psychology.

All in all, Mommy's childhood was a mixture of lollipops, roses and strict discipline. Her fairytale emerged when she married Daddy.

After graduating from secretarial school, Mommy worked at Virginia Mutual Insurance Company in Richmond, Virginia, where she met and became lifelong friends with Hattie Brandon Watson Norrell. "Aunt" Hattie married my mother's uncle Thomas Watson, her mother's youngest brother. She also introduced Mommy to Daddy, Clifton E. Collins Sr.—a brilliant young man in his own right, who started college at the age of sixteen as a math genius. My parents were married as soon as Daddy graduated from college. Aunt Hattie became my oldest brother's godmother.

Mommy gave birth to six kids before beginning work as a bank teller in Syracuse, New York. At that time, my father was serving as a ROTC instructor at Syracuse University. Although I was only around five or six years old at the time, I remember Mommy working at the bank because

Daddy would pile my five brothers and sister into the car to pick Mommy up from work from time to time.

Daddy went to Vietnam twice, and both times, Mommy kept the house together and took great care of us. When I was ten, Mommy worked for the federal government in Fort Knox, Kentucky. When my father started working at Fort Monroe in Virginia, Mommy was transferred to Fort Eustis, about forty-five minutes away. Wanting to always be close together, Mommy applied for an opening on Fort Monroe and got the position. As God would have it, they were assigned to the same organization and worked in the same building. It was a blessing because it meant they could commute together, eat lunch together, shop at the PX or commissary together and have fun flirting with one another through the exchange of glances in the office until it was time for them to go home. This also allowed them to build wonderful relationships with coworkers—connections that were invaluable at a crucial time.

My parents were fun and had many friends. In addition to attending house parties with friends and relatives or throwing parties of their own with delicious food and loud dancing music, Mommy and Daddy belonged to social and civic clubs called Les Femmes and Les Hommes. They were always in good company. In fact, it was in these organizations that they met and socialized with three of the main characters portrayed in the movie Hidden Figures: Katherine Johnson, Dorothy Vaughan, and Mary Jackson.

Mommy's upbringing, her sharp mind, education and ability to adjust to unforeseen challenges played an important role in her ability to run a house like a queen. She had strict policies but was always a warm and caring mother and wife. As a mother, she ran her side of the house, which included my adoring father and six children—four sons, two daughters and a few pets. When I say my mother ran the house, I mean she RAN the house! She got off work, cooked a meal from scratch, checked on her children to see how their day went and made sure Daddy didn't have any worries to provide for us all.

She taught us to respect our father from an early age. As a routine, no matter what we were doing, we were expected to greet Daddy at the door at five-thirty p.m., take his attaché case, present him with his robe and slippers and wait for him to sit down at the table for dinner. We would then ask Daddy if he wanted tea, soda, water or Kool-Aid, ask how many slices of bread he wanted and wait for Mommy to give him his plate. Then Mommy fixed the kids' plates and sat down to eat with us. Daddy always led the prayers, and then we laughed, ate and had caring conversations. If something was wrong in the house, she made sure to bring attention to it, and she and Daddy called a family meeting so we could all learn from the experience.

For as long as I can remember, Mommy always worked—either outside of the house or holding down the fort while Daddy was working or on temporary duty. Extremely ambitious, she loved the challenge of it all. Mommy continued her educational ambitions by taking courses at Elizabethtown Community College in Kentucky and Thomas Nelson Community College in Hampton, Virginia. She was quick witted and articulate in her speech, had a beautiful singing voice and was an extremely talented artist (drawing). She was a fabulous dancer and a superb multitasker and could hang with the best of women and men in friendly debates.

Mommy grew up to be a woman of balance and passed these traits onto her children. We were disciplined, kind, proper, articulate, smart, strong and courageous, and we loved God and Jesus Christ. Mommy and Daddy had a wonderful sense of humor, so we also learned to laugh all the time, especially during challenging moments. We were raised as an upper-middle-class family, surrounded by the best in life. We also knew how to clean a house to perfection, cook delicious meals, take responsibility for jobs and chores and respect and love our parents and others. Sleeping late was never an option if you wanted to make the best of your day, and we always had chores that taught us responsibility early in our lives.

Mommy was our first teacher when it came to English, spelling and philosophy. Daddy was our first math and science teacher. When Mommy was strict, Daddy was soft. When Daddy was strict, Mommy was soft. There was balance.

The whole family was extremely active in sports, and we all learned to adapt to situations quickly and with ease, like most military brats. We moved almost every year for the first fourteen years of my life for Daddy's job in the Army. I didn't mind the moves, because Mommy always made it fun. We were taught it was our duty to move and serve this country, and we needed to stay positive as a show of support for Daddy.

Our parents were role models of what it means to be a supportive member of a family. My parents worked as a team. They never disagreed with each other on issues involving me or my siblings in front of us. They went into their bedroom, closed the door, then come out with the final decision and present this decision together. To this day, out of respect and love, I can honestly say that I never spoke back to my mother or my father and neither have my brothers or sister.

We were raised to believe that the ones who loved us most were God, Jesus, Mommy and Daddy, our sisters and brothers, and our extended family. If we had any problems, we were to go to our parents first then our brothers and sisters, who were many times already in the audience listening to our pleas to Mommy and Daddy. I first experienced and learned about love and affection and how to be all that I could be from my family first. I was allowed to be as strong and as soft as I wanted to be in my family.

I learned how to fix cars, fish, crab, and drive cars and trucks from Daddy, and I learned how to clean a house, grocery shop and cook from my mother. I loved the dual experiences and being Mommy and Daddy's helper. I remember sunny weekend days, sitting under the hood of a car, passing my dad wrenches and screw drivers and then running into the house to help Mommy cook, passing her spatulas and seasonings.

In addition, to Mommy's great looks and a beautiful smile, she was also one of the funniest people I have ever known in my life; her mind was sharp and quick. The great thing and sting about Mommy's humor was that when she was coming for you, she'd sprinkle some truth in everything she said. So, while she was getting you in a debate, full of humor, you learned to laugh at yourself even if the truth stung a little bit. Mommy shared what made you special, as well as your shortcomings. I really enjoyed that.

I loved when she and Daddy got going with each other. Back and forth like a tennis match, teasing and taunting each other in loving ways. Or they'd talk about Mommy's skinny ankles or Daddy's talent of making up words that weren't in the dictionary but made perfect sense. When this form of entertainment began, my brothers, sister and I grabbed a seat on the sofa or floor with popcorn or fruit and watch this loving banter go on for an hour like a primetime television comedy show. I'm not really sure if anyone ever won. I don't think that was the point. We were just seeing a husband and wife, who also happened to be best friends, do what they did best…forget the world and love on each other through down-to-earth clean fun.

My parents believed in always being honest and authentic, no matter what. This meant I grew up telling Mommy and Daddy almost everything! Some things I don't think they really wanted to know. When I was on too much of a roll, they would stop me.

"Janice! We don't want to know everything!"

I didn't know how to lie, and they were my best friends, so my "having diarrhea of the mouth," as Daddy would always say, was part of who I was.

Being the middle child was interesting. No one listens to you because you're stuck in the middle, but on the other hand, because you don't think anyone is listening, you learn to say whatever was on your mind or heart regardless. Why? Because no one is listening. Nonetheless, you know that what you have to say still had value.

Later, I learned my thinking was not exactly accurate. They always listened to me, even though sometimes it didn't appear that way. I talked all the time. Oh boy, could I talk! They each had strategies of engagement when I was on a roll. My mother passively listened to me to make me feel better. She went about the house cleaning, washing and folding clothes and cooking dinner with me on her heels. I talked and talked, expressing myself.

My mother simply said, "Uh huh. Huh. Really? Really? Hmmm."

I loved it!

When I stopped, Mommy asked, "Are you done? Do you feel better?"

"Yes. Thank you, Mommy."

Then I went outside to play, feeling that everything in the world was perfect. I expressed what I had in my heart, Mommy acknowledged my feelings and that was it. She was brilliant with me, as were my brothers who learned to do the same thing.

My older sister Sharon and Daddy were different. They stopped what they were doing and asked me questions the entire time, causing me to get deep sometimes, because someone was listening. I thought maybe they could help me solve all the problems of the world I was facing.

My father often said, "Janice, you're too deep and sensitive at times. Are you okay? Why do you think so much, baby?"

My sister, with the heart and spirit of an artist, would simply say,

"Brilliant, Janice! I love when you express yourself! Write it down. Draw a painting of what you're feeling."

She probably thought I was a little cuckoo…but in our family, cuckoos are loved too! It was great balance having both.

I needed to pull from all these experiences for the next chapter of my life with Mommy.

CHAPTER 2

The Day Things Changed

As you know by now, Mommy was a vibrant, independent, funny, outgoing and incredible woman, wife and mother. She cooked every meal from scratch, washed our clothes, delegated household chores (with six children, why should she do all the work?) and tended to our emotional and pragmatic needs. Selflessness was Mommy's approach, always making sure our needs were met before hers. A role model of self-pride, she always looked nice when she went out in public.

She told me, "Janice, remember you're a Collins, and you never know who you'll run into at the grocery store. So, dress like you're somebody."

My mother also believed in having an active voice. She was very opinionated and outspoken—we all were in our family; it was an expectation.

All this changed in 1995.

In 1995, my mother had a stroke. One Wednesday afternoon, one of my father's sisters, Aunt Delores, was visiting from New York, so they decided to go to one of my mother's favorite shops in Phoebus, Virginia. Mommy had purchased quite a few collector's dolls from this special shop over the years.

After parking, Daddy went around to Mommy's side to assist her out of the truck. (Daddy always opened the door for Mommy and buckled her seatbelt going in and opened Mommy's door and took her seatbelt off when they got to their destination. Talk about chivalry!)

When Mommy got out of the truck, she stumbled. She assured Daddy she was okay, but he watched her. They made jokes about it and kept going as usual.

When they got to the front porch of the doll store, Mommy chose to sit on the porch rather than go inside. This was weird. Daddy felt something was wrong, but he wasn't sure what it was. He didn't make a big deal out of it, but he was worried. He watched her from inside the store as she remained seated on the porch, never going in. I can only imagine what Mommy was feeling or thinking as the stroke started to settle in. I'm sure she didn't know what was going on exactly, but she knew something wasn't right.

The next morning, Daddy noticed that Mommy was quieter than normal. He went into action and took her to the doctor. She couldn't see her primary doctor who had been seeing her for almost thirty years. The doctor on duty surmised that she had a bad cold and would get better. That was on a Thursday. Almost a week and a half later, my brothers Ronald and Donald, their wives Tameka and Gabrielle, and my sister Sharon—all in the medical field—had taken her vitals and began assessing her.

At the time, I was working at a television station in Atlanta, Georgia. I spoke to Mommy on the phone.

"Hey, baby! How are you doing?" Mommy asked.

"I'm good, Mommy. How are you? Daddy tells me that you're not feeling well. What's going on?"

"Girl, I don't know. Hey, baby! How are you doing?"

"I'm good, Mommy. What's going on?"

"I'm fine. Hey, baby! How are you doing?" Mommy asked me for the third time.

I immediately knew something was wrong, so I asked Mommy to please put Daddy back on the phone. "Daddy, something's not right. Mommy needs to go to the doctor immediately."

For my entire life, Mommy never, ever repeated herself. She said something once, so you needed to listen well and attentively. Mommy had taught us another lesson—how to listen and understand…something was definitely wrong.

Daddy took her to her primary doctor, Dr. Ollie T. Adcock. It took Dr. Adcock less than ten minutes to diagnose that Mommy had suffered a stroke. Immediately, an ambulance was called to take her to Riverside Hospital in Newport News, Virginia, where Mommy and Daddy stayed together for nine days.

I caught a flight quickly out of Atlanta to see them. When I walked into the room, Mommy was up, bright, energetic, and said, "Hey, baby."

But her eye movements and the raising of her left arm to wave was a little slow. By the fifth day in the hospital, Mommy had lost the use of her left side. Had the stroke been diagnosed earlier, perhaps the damage would not have been as serious. Instead, the bleeding continued in both sides of her brain. I stayed with Mommy every day of my visit. I remember precious moments when Mommy looked at me and smiled, but she didn't speak. The stroke was still manifesting itself.

One night, she struggled to get to sleep for hours. I asked, "Mommy are you tired?"

"Yes."

"Would you like to go to sleep?"

"Yes."

"Okay, watch me. Close your eyes like this." As I demonstrated, she closed her eyes and went to sleep.

Another precious moment was when I began to sing. My mother and sister are the real singers in the family. I'm what they call the entertainer, who can slide through some notes with feeling. I sang *His Eye Was on the Sparrow*. I didn't know if it was to comfort me or Mommy, but she smiled and closed her eyes, drifting off to sleep.

At the end of nine days in the hospital, Mommy was transported to the Riverside Rehabilitation Facility in Hampton, Virginia, where she stayed for five and a half weeks. Daddy stayed with her the whole time in the rehabilitation center, 24/7. He had them declare her room private and secured an Army cot with an air mattress as his bed. Through every aspect of her stay—dining, exercising, speech therapy and occupational therapy—he accompanied Mommy, providing all her personal needs, such as bathing. He never wanted her to feel alone, paying attention to the small details like pushing her wheelchair along the waterfront of the Chesapeake Bay for fresh air and a change of scenery that didn't say "hospital." Daddy said you never know what a person really means to you until a tragedy occurs. He considered it a blessing to be able to care of every need Mommy had through all the challenges.

Like my father, I also felt it was a blessing to care for Mommy—even if it was long distance. In the few months after Mommy had the stroke, I called her every single day to check on her, to hear her voice and to check on Daddy as well. I flew home every month to "put my eyes on her," as we say when we need to settle our nerves and spirit. These monthly visits to see my mother did not bring peace to my heart, because I always returned to Atlanta. I felt like I could do more—that my parents really needed me. I continued to pray. God doesn't work in confusion.

One day after prayer, my heart was lifted. The answer emerged. Since living and working in Atlanta was not bringing me peace at this time, I decided to move back to Virginia permanently. I was the only one in my family who wasn't married or had children, so it made logistical sense. It also just felt right, without confusion or worry. I knew it was the right answer from God.

Suddenly, my heart was at peace, settled, and with a smile on my face, I packed my bags, put my career on hold, drove home and became a fulltime caregiver for my mother. The day I decided to leave my job as a newscast producer at WXIA in Atlanta to move home to Virginia, great things were happening for me. I had just received a sizable raise, won some more Emmys, and while I didn't have a job waiting for me, I knew in my heart this was the best decision. Now, a little over twenty years later, I can honestly say I have no regrets about my choice. It was the best thing I ever did, not just for my mother and family, but for myself as well.

Obvious changes were omnipresent. Mommy didn't cook anymore or engage in household chores or even delegate. She didn't laugh and hardly spoke, but when she did, she whispered. The simple things she used to do so naturally—like walking, washing herself, going to the bathroom by herself—were no longer easy or even doable. She no longer danced when a good song came on. Because she was so strong and independent, it had always been hard for her to ask someone for help. Imagine the challenge she faced with this now.

In addition to physical challenges, emotional despair hung in the balance as well. The possibility of despair, fear, anger, sadness, uncertainty, lack of confidence, embarrassment, helplessness and shame became a part of Mommy's everyday way of life for a time. But it was well hidden for the most part. Still, these emotions lay before her to choose. Key word: choose.

From the moment Mommy woke up to the time she was relaxed enough to go to sleep, she had to learn to live with it all. The good news was she didn't face any of this alone. The entire immediate and extended family pitched in to do whatever was necessary to get her through. Mommy decided to take it one day at a time.

You may be going through something like this yourself. If you are, hang in there. It can get better.

During those years, I was honored to care for my mother (and in many ways, my father). She and I grew to be the best of friends. She admired me as the weird, odd-ball daughter who was unpredictable at times, doing things Mommy couldn't do like ride a motorcycle or work on my '69 Chevy. She thought I was cool and bold. Our whole family was close, but now Mommy and I became closer than ever before.

At the same time, you probably know that being close is not always good! But there are lessons to be learned from the change in proximity and meaning. I'll get into that later. For now, let me say that caregiving can be challenging for the survivor and the giver, and the last time I checked, there aren't a lot of books on how to get through the trials with humor. Well, this is that book, a story about how we made it through, pragmatically and strategically, with an added dose of humor.

Mommy and I are sharing this journey with you, so perhaps you can find some moments of laughter while facing the challenges of surviving and thriving after a stroke. From Mommy calling everything tangible "chicken" to her relearning how to speak with her authentic voice that had been shoved to another place in her brain, through her love and faith in God, her love for her husband and family and her great sense of humor, Mommy began living again!

She laughed, cooked, danced and shimmied her way through one of the hardest fights of her life. The fight to stay positive, the will to win and the spirituality to laugh loudly in the face of her opponent…the almighty stroke!

CHAPTER 3

It's a Long Way to Z

Mommy was in rehabilitation for almost six weeks. It's like learning the ABCs all over again. It's a long way to Z when you're starting over from the basics. Many times, you and your caregiver may feel the struggle of every single letter, so expect frustration, sadness, depression, anger and even a giving-up attitude from time to time. With an attitude of perseverance, you can also expect happy times!

In occupational therapy, every day brought challenges, but Mommy never gave up. Her initial task was to put small, plastic blocks into shaped holes. The first day, Mommy couldn't do it. Out of frustration, she threw a block across the room. "I can't do it."

For the rest of the session that day, Mommy did a lot of yelling and throwing blocks. Being my silly self, I turned it into a sporting game and tried to catch the blocks she was throwing with my mouth. I finally caught one (they were small).

"Ah hah!" I yelled with enthusiasm. "And you thought I couldn't catch it!"

The mood lightened up, which gave Mommy a little more energy to keep trying.

"Come on, Mommy! Try again! You can do it!" I said to her with confidence and reassurance.

When Tuesday rolled around, Mommy got closer to fitting a block into its appropriate hole but kept missing it, despite her exhausting efforts.

"Hey, it's only Tuesday. Keep trying!"

Mommy looked at me kind of sadly. She was trying to adjust to how the stroke had affected her. She was frustrated and nervous and wondered if she would ever be able to do *normal* things again.

On Wednesday, Mommy did it! She got one out of four! Yay! We both danced in our seats.

"You got one! You got one!" I shouted.

Thursday rolled around, and Mommy got three out of four correct. This time, we stood up together, shook our hips, hugged and kept saying, "Yes! Yes! Yes!"

"Did you see that, Janice?" Mommy asked with enthusiasm and pride.

"I sure did! You got this, Mommy!"

Friday was finally here, and we were confident and nervous at the same time. I think this feeling is normal. You win one race, then a second, then you want to try out for the Olympics! She had done so well and kept improving; we wondered what the day would bring.

Three hours went by. Mommy took her time, concentrated and moved with confidence. Then … Mommy got four holes in one! She got all four blocks correctly into their appropriate holes in one session!

"Yay! I knew you could do it, Mommy! I knew you could do it!"

"I did it! I did it! I did it!" Mommy shouted.

We all celebrated—including the therapist—with hugging, moving our hips and letting out cheers. It was great!

It's good to remember that time, patience and perseverance are keys to achieving optimal results in rehabilitation. At the end, through hard work and being consistent, it's all worth it.

If there's regression, which will happen from time to time, shake it off. Remember, you've done it before, and you can do it again. So, keep at it!

Another key is learning to recognize and address fear. Many times, fear is either in the spotlight or on the periphery of every situation.

Early on in Mommy's therapy, when she was doing physical therapy on her stomach on the mat, she'd sometimes scream like she was in pain.

"Come on, Mrs. Collins. Get up on your knees. You can do it. Come on," said the therapist.

"Aaagggggghhhhhhh," Mommy yelled.

"Can you roll yourself over, Mrs. Collins?"

"Aauuuggghhhh," Mommy yelled out again.

"You can do it, Mrs. Collins."

"Aauuggghhhhh!"

I watched Mommy do this over and over and over during physical therapy. When I took a closer look, I noticed there weren't any tears when she screamed, and it didn't appear as if she was in pain. She had a safety belt wrapped around her waist, and the therapists were trying to get her to push herself up from the mat onto her knees. Each time they grabbed her belt to help her, she'd scream. Sometimes she screamed before they even touched her or the belt. I knew there was more to this than what met the eyes and ears! It was fear—and not just her own fear; she was implanting fear in others.

After watching her for a few days, I figured it out. Mommy was afraid of hurting herself when she tried to do something she had been doing without any help for fifty-seven years. She was acting like this to scare the therapists, so she wouldn't have to do the exercises.

I laughed inside and thought, "Hhmm, how clever."

Mommy needed this physical therapy, so I decided to do something about it. The trick was figuring out how to get her to do the exercise while addressing the fear she might be feeling and make sure she didn't hurt herself. I came up with a plan.

At our next therapy session, when Mommy was in the middle of one of her screaming arias on the mat, I got on the floor with her. I laid down next to her and stared. Every time she screamed, I was right there staring at her, straight into her eyes. She screamed a few more times when they asked her to get up on her knees. I just laid there and stared. Probably needing a break from the screaming, the therapists walked away for a few minutes. I continued staring at her. Finally, she stopped and stared back at me. I began a conversation.

"Hey, Mommy," I whispered.

"Hi."

"Can I ask you something?"

"What?"

"Why are you screaming?"

"I don't know." She started laughing.

"Well, you have to be screaming for some reason. Why are you screaming?"

"Because I'm scared I might hurt myself."

"Have you hurt yourself yet?"

"No."

I made a face, and we laughed at that answer.

"So, listen. Will you do me a small favor today?"

"What?" she asked.

"Can you not scream unless you really have to? Because I'm starting to go a little *deaf*." For effect, I added loudly, "Okay?"

She laughed. "Okay."

"I also know that you sometimes scream to scare them, hoping they'll leave you alone. Good idea, but why don't you save that screaming for something really, really hard. Okay?"

She paused "Okay, yeah, that'll work."

I replied, "Now can you please try and roll over without screaming? I'll help you."

Mommy giggled. "Okay."

And a rollin' she went. Whew! It wasn't easy, but we did it, and there was no screaming. Every time she formed her mouth like she was going to scream, I gave her a look that read, "Don't you dare."

Then we went back to work. We did it! Then we laid out on our backs and just laughed. It felt good to succeed and not get hurt.

Another time Mommy had to face fear was when she was getting off an airport shuttle bus, approximately two years after her stroke. Daddy got off the shuttle first and turned to help her. She was shaking and screaming lightly in small bursts, afraid to take the last step off the shuttle. People were patiently waiting, wanting to catch their flights. They could have been mean and impatient, but they just watched and waited.

Each time Mommy tried to step down, she'd scream because she was afraid of what could happen with one wrong step.

It's difficult to have faith in a body, or even a foot, that doesn't want to obey your brain and may not be as strong as it used to be. It makes sense to be afraid. When this happens, it may be helpful to learn how to lean on others and trust them. Sometimes all one needs is reassurance.

I continued standing there, watching as she put her left foot out—the one the stroke affected—and then pull it back in. Then out again and back. Out and back. Out and back. I realized she was doing the hokey pokey without the chorus or music. Now that I think about it, singing that song might have helped her get off the bus. But, at the time, we had Daddy, and he was great.

Daddy stepped in (no pun intended, but funny). "Come on, baby. I got you."

"I'm coming. I'm coming…auuuggghhhh," Mommy yelled because she was nervous.

She also didn't like a lot of attention, especially this kind where she was stopping others from getting off the shuttle—something that was letting others know she was different.

At this point, it was easier for Mommy to move forward rather than turn around and get back on the shuttle. Physically, that would have been extremely difficult.

She never gave up. With everything going on, she continued her hardest to take that extra step. Five minutes passed, and the hokey pokey continued, as well as the bursts of screams. Left foot out. Left foot in.

"Auuugghhh!"

"Calm down, baby. I got you. You're doing great!" Daddy's constant reassurance was so beautiful and amazing. He was so patient.

"I'm coming. I promise. Please don't rush me, Cliff," Mommy pleaded.

Left leg went out, back in, out, in. Fifteen minutes passed. "I promise. I'm coming!"

Twenty minutes passed. Mommy had gone through instances like this before. As much as she wanted to do some things herself, sometimes, she'd get a little stuck. The fear and physical challenges combined made everything that was once easy seem hard, if not impossible.

But Daddy was great. The other passengers were great, and we all waited patiently. We never yelled at her. Instead, we used patience, and the subtle mention of a deadline.

"Baby, try one more time. Then I'm going to help you. Okay?" my father gently said.

"Okay." Left leg went out and in again.

"Come on, baby." Daddy lifted Mommy up and off the shuttle. "You did wonderful, baby."

"Thank you, Cliff. I was sooooo scared."

"I know, baby. Don't worry. You did wonderful. Now let's go catch our flight. Okay?"

"Okay."

They kissed, everyone clapped, we waved and said thank you. We were off to catch our flight to Florida, then a cruise to Alaska.

Riding the Rainbow

The lessons of this story are patience, patience, patience. If you can, get into all forms of therapy immediately and put the work in. Never give up and know that kindness in others is not only beautiful, but it's also another part of therapy. Soak it all in, and when things get rough or they get stuck, sometimes you must get them moving forward any way you can. Just be careful not to hurt them or yourself and always try to be encouraging.

CHAPTER 4

NOOOOOOOOO...ZZZZZZEEEEEYYYYYY

After someone has a stroke, there can be noticeable changes in their personality. Some personality traits become exaggerated. More pronounced. More intense. Although you *may* see the change, the person who has had the stroke may not . . . until it's too late.

Pre-stroke, Mommy was . . . let's say, inquisitive. No, no, let's say curious. No, that doesn't fit either. Let's be honest and say she could be sssssssooooooo nnnnooooosssszzzzzzzzzeeeeeyyyyy at times! A very protective mother of six children, she was always on the lookout for safety issues when it came to the environment around her children.

Reading lips, body language, facial expressions, mail left on the table . . . I'm kidding about that last one. But you get the idea. She was always on the lookout for things that could hurt us, whether it was an object, a person or something happening. This meant that she had her eyes and ears open and at an attention!

After Mommy's stroke, if we were ever out in public... everything was fair game and let me tell you, my mother's ears were fine-tuned and skilled like a bat! In fact, a bat had nothing on her nicely shaped ears. Going into a crowded restaurant--boy oh boy!!! It was open season! It was like CNN, NBC, ABC, CBS AND the BBC all rolled up into one! An informative arena with gossip coming from every direction . . . a positively thrilling day for Mommy!

Like the time Mommy and I went out to eat at a local restaurant.

"Okay, Mommy. I know it's going to be hard but try and concentrate on eating your food."

"Okay," she replied.

I caught her rolling her eyes at the fact that her daughter was telling her what to do. I laugh now, thinking about what she really wanted to tell me. Anyway, we got seated, and I began catching her up on the latest soap opera happenings.

"Jack is really angry, but not as angry as Victor." I never watched soap operas until I started taking care of Mommy and grew to love the juicy stories. It was a special time between the two of us.

As I spoke, she stared straight at me as though she was paying close attention to every single word I said.

"Well, Victor and Nikki were at it again," I continued. I noticed Mommy leaning to her right. "Mommy, are you listening or are you being nosey"?

"No, go ahead. I'm listening."

Our waitress made her way to our table. "Are you ready to order?"

"Yes, I'll have the turkey salad with crackers and tea, please. Thank you."

The waitress then turned to Mommy. "And you, ma'am?"

Mommy was leaning so far that her hair was almost in a woman's plate at the table next to us! When the woman looked down to fork up some broccoli, she noticed Mommy's head and started to laugh!

"Mommy! I caught you! You're being nosey!"

"No, I'm not!"

"Then how did you get mashed potatoes in your hair?"

We both laughed hysterically. Mommy had tuned into a conversation that was too hard to resist and didn't realize how far she was leaning into it.

No one got hurt, and it was a good laugh. From the medical perspective, it was an over exaggeration of a gesture, because her mind didn't adjust for the depth perception.

Riding the Rainbow

If something like this happens to you, try not to be upset or embarrassed. The survivors of a stroke are doing the best that they can, and sometimes things happen without them knowing it.

We were lucky with Mommy, because she was always funny, even before the stroke. Some things may have changed, but some things stayed the same, and we were grateful.

CHAPTER 5

A Shopping We Will Go

Before Mommy had her stroke, she used to go grocery shopping for the entire family. Daddy pushed the buggy, and she made the selections. She ran a very tight ship. In fact, growing up, people often commented on how well-mannered her children were at the commissary or any store. Before going into a store, Mommy gave the orders. "I have a list, and we are going to follow this list and get all that we need. Nothing else."

To control all six of us, Mommy had us form a line and hold each other's hands—from the oldest to the youngest, with Mommy at the front. We smiled and spoke when spoken to, so Mommy could concentrate on the task at hand and not worry about us running off. We did exactly what we were told to do entering the store, while shopping and when exiting.

Budgeting while shopping with her was a valuable lesson; "wants" are less important than "needs" when on a budget. We learned to be grateful for what we had, and we never wanted or asked for anything. We had the blessing of good health and nice clothes. We grew up in a nice house in a nice neighborhood and had plenty of food to eat. All that came from Mother and Father. Nothing was missed, including our parents always knowing what we wanted. We were given gifts when affordable and age appropriate.

After the stroke, not being able to walk around freely made Mommy a bit nervous. Like the day she went shopping with my sister Sharon and decided to use one of those shopping cart automobiles. We fondly call them sports cars. One time, she almost ended up in the meat department. Literally! Mommy was going so fast in her sports car that when she ran into a low-to-the-ground meat selection container, the cart tipped like it was going to dump her right into the bin! Once my sister made sure Mommy was okay, they had a good laugh.

Well, now it was my turn to shop with Mommy, and I looked at it as a fun field trip. As soon as we got to the grocery store and the car was parked, I raced inside to get one of the sports cars. I turned the handle to see how much speed it had and then jumped in and raced to the car, trying not to take the curve too sharply and topple the thing.

When Mommy saw me, she laughed. "Janice, you are so crazy! You're a fool!"

Great, I thought to myself! *The first iceberg is broken. Mommy isn't nervous.*
"Okay, Mommy, let's do this!"

Sharon usually did the shopping, so I went through a quick tutorial on how the cart worked with Mommy, and off we went. I ran ahead of Mommy to stop traffic to let the queen pass. She started off a little hesitant, but then started to speed up. I saw her smiling as she began to get used to it.

As we made our way across the parking lot, I stopped parking lot traffic to allow for safe passage and lightly jogged behind Mommy as she enjoyed her new form of freedom. I called out commands.

"Gas! . . . brake! . . . gas! . . . brake! . . . slow down, Mommy! Brake! . . . gas!"

Whew! We made it inside the store. Safe.

"Okay, I have the list. Let's go," I said confidently.

Mommy smiled and leaned to her left a bit, being cool, with a little 'gangsta' lean, you might call it. Well, let me tell you. By the time we got through the shopping list, Mommy was flying! Then soaring in her sports car! Boy was it fun!

I loved it, even when my feet started to get tired. I asked Mommy to give me a lift . . . all 200 pounds of me on that little, itty-bitty cart.

She laughed when I jumped on the side. "Lord, Janice, you're going to tip this thing over!"

Nonetheless, we kept on rolling. Down the aisles. Up the aisles. Sometimes almost on two wheels (not a good idea), but it was liberating for both of us. Our nervousness diminished with every successful turn of the wheel and corner.

Being confident, Mommy returned to her normal shopping self but loaded up on more than the groceries. She took a corner so fast and sharp, she hooked a woman's purse and kept going! She laughed as I ran after her yelling. "Put on the brake! Brake!"

She picked up a corner rack as well! And what was Mommy doing? Did she panic? Nope! She was going, "WWWWWEEEEEEEEEEEEEE!!!!!!!," and laughing uncontrollably!

"Mommy! Hit the brakes!"

Because Mommy was laughing so hard, she couldn't put on the brakes. Too much was going on for her brain to balance it all. Her brain wouldn't allow her to do two things at once.

"The brakes! The brakes," I yelled like Tattoo from Fantasy Island.

Finally, she rotated her wrist and came to a stop. I was calling out the wrong instructions when I told her to hit the brakes, but she pulled it all together, and we all had a good laugh. Thank goodness it was plastic utensils on the rack she picked up along the way, and the woman was very sweet and laughed with us when we returned her purse to her.

Now, something to keep in mind. After practice and repetition, Mommy's brain adjusted. In many ways, she began to react as quickly as her mind worked and as quickly as her eyes could see, which both were still as sharp as thumbtacks in some ways.

If Mommy saw something she liked and could reach it, it was in the basket. This meant that the short grocery list transformed into a long list of add-ons. But that was perfectly fine. Everything was trying to get back to normal.

To the checkout line we went.

"Your total is fifty-two dollars, ma'am," the cashier said.

Mommy got $60 out of her wallet with a little assistance from me. She received the change, handed it to me, and I put it into her wallet. All was well.

"Ready to go?"

"Yes!" she screamed with excitement.

She knew it was over, and she had done well. She was proud of herself and so was I. We zzzzzzzooooooooommmmmeeeeddddd across the parking lot and to the car. When she got in, Mommy kissed me on the cheek. "Thank you, Janice."

I looked at her. "We owe a lot to Sharon and Daddy, Mommy. They are the ones who helped get you started on shopping! It was a lot of fun, and you are very welcome, pardner!"

By the time I got the sports car back to its rightful location, no one could tell it had gone on a special trip with us. Special indeed.

Riding the Rainbow

Going shopping and encouraging their freedom and their freedom of choice and independence are well worth any price, even at the checkout line. When paying with a check, or signing of a document in general, if at all possible, let them sign their own name, even if you have to help them a bit by placing your hand over theirs to help them write.

If they're paying by cash, still allow them to participate to the best of their ability. It was difficult for Mommy to sign her checks with her signature, because the stroke had affected her left-hand, her dominant hand. She had the most beautiful handwriting before the stroke.

One day, my younger brother Michael, who is a natural artist, was working with Mommy on drawing and discovered that if she closed her eyes and imagined and remembered what her signature looked like, with her eyes closed and using her right hand, she could write her signature almost flawlessly! Amazing right? From that point on, when Mommy needed to sign her name, she'd closed her eyes, used her right hand, and signed . . . beautifully!

CHAPTER 6

The Freedom Rides

Sometimes, it's all about freedom and being outdoors. The hardest part is the first step or the first push on the gas.

"Hey, Mommy, let's go for a ride," I said with excitement.

"I don't want to," she replied.

I knew she wasn't being honest, because she was always ready to go for a ride. She just didn't want to go down the stairs of our split-level house.

"Come on. It's a great day! A beautiful day! We need to get outside."

I sat and waited, and sat and waited, and talked a bit. I sat and waited some more.

I talked to Mommy calmly, and after about an hour, I finally talked her into moving. Actually, I don't think I talked her into anything. I think she made up her mind to do it–especially if it meant shutting me up.

We made it safely down the stairs and into the car.

"Thank you, God. Thank you, Jesus. I made it! That's nothing but the Lord, Janice! Did you know that? Do you hear me girlfriend?" Mommy loved to accomplish things, especially when they were extremely challenging and frightful—always acknowledging the presence from whom all blessings flow.

"Yep, you and the Lord, Mommy. Let's go."

Mommy buckled up, and I pulled slowly out of the driveway.

I shouted, "Hang on!"

That's something I've always done whenever we got in a car . . . like we were at the starting line at the Grand Prix or Indy 500. This always got her excited. Mommy's head jerked back onto the seat as I took off with a look of determination on my face like a Speed Racer animation coming to life. She giggled and smiled as I raced down the street.

Getting out was the best part. That was it. Getting out into the world with other people. Out into the sunshine. Watching people, cars and birds go by. We drove around town looking at what the world had to offer: the beautiful waters on the peninsula, the beaches and the magnificent Hampton Coliseum.

We decided to stay outside for lunch. We grabbed a box lunch, parked at a nearby park and ate in front of a lake. Nice and relaxing. After taking my last bite, I looked at Mommy and smiled.

"What, Janice?" she asked nervously.

"Now, it's your turn."

"My turn for what?" She realized what I was about to do—better yet, what *she* was about to do!

She said, "Oh sh—" (we never said the whole word, but you knew what was meant).

"Come on. You can still drive, right?"

"Oh sh—," she said again and again. Her license had been taken away after the stroke.

"Listen, I can take care of you if something happens, but you have to also be able to take care of me, okay?"

"Oh sh—," she continued to say.

I laughed, excited about what was to come. I quickly raced to her side of the car and got her out of the car. We danced our way back to the driver's side. I gently sat her in the hot seat—I mean driver's seat—and buckled her in. And, yes, she was still saying, "Oh sh—, oh sh—."

I felt the energy of excitement in the car rise. Mommy was smiling but was still terribly nervous.

I got into the passenger's seat and tried my best to get my hands and feet in positions of safety in case I needed to quickly help out. (Sidenote: this would have been a great time to have a driver's ed double steering wheel and pedals car for survivors of strokes. Oh well, we made do.)

"Okay, Mommy, let's go. No one's in the parking lot. It's you, me and some trees . . . so try not to hit them." I lightly giggled while Mommy just sat there nervous, not moving.

It was all over her face, but she also smiled with anticipation. I laughed the whole time but only on the inside. After realized what I had said and done, I got a little nervous, too.

What am I thinking? What was I thinking? Was I thinking? Oh, Lord! Is this a good idea?

Suddenly, Mommy yelled out, "Hang on!"

My head jerked back, and I said, "Oh sh—!"

And just like that, Mommy was driving around an empty parking lot. Just she and I and the trees…which she did not hit. Not one. I smiled as I watched Mommy drive for the first time in years. Around and around and around in circles, she was driving . . . flawlessly. Brake, gas, brake, gas . . . like she was driving cross country. Wow! And they said she couldn't drive!

My heart began to warm up, and I smiled. The car was filled with achievement, love and happiness. I didn't say one word while she was driving because I didn't want to distract her or make her nervous. I also didn't speak because I didn't want to be distracted or nervous either! <laughing>

"Look! Look, everyone! I'm driving," Mommy yelled. "I'm driving!"

It was such a great ride. She was so happy just driving around an empty parking lot. That moment served as a beautiful reminder that wonderful things can happen in small places and spaces. Seize the moment, take the opportunity and, for heaven's sake, make sure there aren't any cars or people around! <laughing>

Mommy brought the car to a stop, put it into park, then looked at me—still smiling—and stuck her tongue out. This was her way of saying, "See, I told you I could do it."

It was also her way of saying thank you.

"Now that was a great ride," I said.

Mommy said, "No sweat. No big deal."

No BIG DEAL?! Riiiggghht. She couldn't stop talking about it for a week. The first call she made was to her sister Jackey.

"Hey, Jackey!"

"Hey, Vi!"

"Guess what?" Mommy said.

"What?"

"I went driving today! Janice took me driving. I mean, I drove. I drove! I had her swinging around the car like she does me!"

Aunt Jackey laughed heartily on the other end of the phone. It was wonderful to hear them laughing and sharing a special moment together.

It's always good to do things to remind the survivor and caregiver that, in a lot of ways, the survivor is still the same person and can still do some of the same things. Explore the possibilities. You'll be glad to know that things haven't totally changed.

It was a great day.

Then there were THE DRIVES. These happened on a regular basis.

Daddy came home. "Hey, baby."

"Hey," Mommy responded.

"It sure is a nice night. Come on," Daddy said.

Mommy trusted Daddy, and she confidently and excitedly proceeded down the stairs with him. No questions asked.

Okay, so he had to give her a few kisses to convince her it was going to be okay, but it worked like a charm—as charming as Daddy has always been. They were lovebirds before the stroke and were lovebirds after the stroke as well. It was all good.

They got in Daddy's red Dakota truck and headed out for a romantic drive. They drove around parks and fountains and across Hampton Roads Bridge with Wilson Pickett playing in the background on a cassette tape. Like teenagers, they even stopped for ice cream. Mommy felt sixteen all over again. Okay, maybe eighteen. No, twenty-one. Yeah, they met when she was twenty-one.

My dad did a fabulous job of keeping the romance going as much as possible, and my mom loved every bit of it. Mommy knew what to expect for Saturday mornings. They hit the road. Shopping. Eating out at restaurants. Going to the movies or short weekend trips. You name it.

After being out for hours, Daddy laid Mommy's seat back, so she could rest as they made their way home.

"Baby, are you ready to go in yet? We've had a full day of driving?" Daddy asked Mommy.

Mommy suddenly sat up, fully awake. "No!"

Daddy laughed and kept on driving. They began at noon and drove until almost ten at night before they finally made it home.

I watched from the hallway as Daddy prepared Mommy for bed, helping put her pajamas on.

She looked at Daddy. "Thank you, baby."

Dad replied, "You're welcome, baby. Did you have fun?"

Mommy exclaimed, "Yes! Yes! Yes, I did!" And right then, at that moment, Mommy was like a new woman. Ready for another ride.

"Janice, Janice, jahnneeeesssee," Mommy called out. "Guess what?"

I said, "What's up, shortay?"

"We just got in. We went everywhere. You young people can't keep up with us!"

I conceded graciously. "I know, Mommy. We can't keep up."

We all laughed, and I thanked God for a daddy like the Daddy we were blessed with, as I headed to my room to rest for the night, in peaceful sleep.

Riding the Rainbow

Now, you tell me. From reading this story, do you think Mommy felt alive AND was living her best life? You betcha! So, get out there and take a ride!

It may be a bit challenging to get survivors of strokes outdoors, but once you do, wait until you try and get them back inside! It doesn't always have to be a drive. Sitting outside in the sun, soaking up vitamin D can be enjoyable as well.

CHAPTER 7

It's the Small Things

I want you to think of how magnets come together for a moment. When two magnets are brought close together, they connect if one is positive and the other is negative. The force of magnetism allows two opposite energy forces to connect. This equation can be used when dealing with the aftermath of strokes.

After someone has a stroke, they usually face some type of physical limitation. This is the negative. While the physical limitation is visible on the outside of the person stricken with the stroke, deep inside, they still want to do the same physical things they once did. That desire is still there. That desire, that emotion, is the positive.

The next step is to find creative ways of bringing the physical challenges and the emotional desires together for movement to drive the recovery train forward. This can be tricky but not impossible. It's best to spend time identifying emotional obstacles that may stop forward movement. The person affected by the stroke may be embarrassed about how their bodies move differently or perhaps they're sad and depressed because they don't move the same way. Or sometimes, they don't move anymore because they don't think they can. They can't stand up for very long, much less head down the Soul Train Line or play the air guitar while they're dancing like they used to. In these situations, I believe in having a party—movement—right where they're sitting!

One day as Mommy sat on the side of the bed watching music videos, I noticed she was moving her shoulders a little. She had always been a fantastic dancer. I was ready!

"Go, Mommy! Go, Mommy! Now left, now left, now right, now right."

Mommy's shoulders were moving. She was dancing.

"And shake it! Shake it! Shake it! Do the worm! Do the worm! Do the Bankhead bounce! Do the Bankhead bound! Now bounce! Bounce! Bounce!" I was really getting into it and calling out instructions until we both burst out laughing! It was fun and got Mommy moving and doing something she always loved–dancing. This blessing happened because I didn't look at what she couldn't do but at what she *could* do, right from where she was sitting.

Exercise of the body, mind, spirit and emotion are all important. If they danced before, they'll still want to dance after the stroke. Believe me, even if they can't do the same moves, their spirit tries and can adjust to their new bodies and their new dance.

Here's a little secret as a bonus. Sometimes their caregiver, who's cheering them on and calling out the moves, needs to keep it to themselves that dancing is a form of exercise. Shhh…using the word *exercise* can take the fun out of it!

One day when we were on a trip out of town, Al Green was playing on the radio when Daddy came back to the hotel room. Mommy said to him, "Baby, remember the parties we used to go to, in the basement?" Wink, wink.

My mother could be so frisky sometimes. Daddy blushed. "Ah hey hey hey, yeah baby, I remember. Come on, baby. Let's dance." He helped Mommy stand, and they danced together.

In the comfort of his secure embrace, she moved a little bit more, almost like doing the worm. Her spirit was dancing and then so was she. Daddy held her up, holding her tightly, and they swayed and danced together, like they'd done a thousand times before. I watched my parents as they fell in love all over again. It was a wonderful sight to see as I lay across the bed watching the two of them.

And to think, dancing after the stroke began with me coming into Mommy's room one day, dancing to a song she liked. Before that time, once Mommy had the stroke, she had stopped dancing. She didn't think she could or should. She thought that, in a very interesting way, she needed to *act* like she had a stroke. I imagine that meant not doing things she had always done. Wrong!

It's important to stop trying to fit in when God wants you to stand out! Stand out and away from the stroke to return to who you are. In this spirit, once the seal of getting back to normalcy had been broken, Mommy danced whenever she felt it and kept dancing whenever she could, wherever she could and however she could.

One thing to remember is that while the stroke survivor may love dancing in the privacy of their own homes, they may not be ready to dance in public. You know, around other people. The survivor may be a little paranoid about how they look to other people. They may think they look uncoordinated or clumsy. So, as you encourage your loved one, consider practicing at home first. Then introduce them to the world and the world to them again. Stay close to them and dance every chance you get.

Oh yeah, one more thing. If they are used to singing, help them to return to this gift. Mommy had a beautiful talking and singing voice. She liked to sing in the car, her room, in the living room—it didn't matter.

I got Mommy to sing again by singing for the *shows*—the drag shows, that is. Right in her bedroom. It started one day when Mommy and I were in her room talking. I told her about a drag show I saw in person or on television. I imitated how the drag queens lip synced, exaggerating the vibration of a silent and false falsetto, swing my make-believe Cher-hair, and smile as wide as Diana Ross in Central Park. Mommy laughed so hard at how silly I was acting.

Mommy couldn't help herself. She had to join in on the fun. We took turns. We played a fabulous song, Mommy sang and I was the drag queen lip synching her words. Then we switched. I sang and Mommy lip synched the songs. Oh, my goodness, we really loved this game!

This was another unexpected blessing that brought Mommy and I closer. It also brought us to tears with laughter, got the lungs and body moving, along with a nice boost of confidence. Here's to all the fabulous drag queens around the world who helped play a role in Mommy's recovery. Yes! And twirl! And twirl! Now drop!

Riding the Rainbow

Remember, it's not just getting there that's important. It's also *the way you get them there* that can make the healing process and life enjoyable once again. So, sing, dance and twirl. From that first step, that first note, Mommy never stopped dancing and singing, and neither should you.

CHAPTER 8

Stories from El Cuatro de Bano

Every day, there are challenges, and sometimes, instead of dealing with these challenges, Mommy tried to avoid them for as long as possible. It's kind of like imposing a self-induced act of torture that I'd have to pull her back from whenever possible. Mommy's self-induced acts of torture were made evident during one of our road trips.

After hours of riding in the car, I said, "Mommy, do you have to use the bathroom?"

"No," she quickly answered.

I knew how much water she drank that day, so I knew she needed to use the bathroom. I imagined what was going on inside Mommy's head. Each time I questioned her, the word yes flashed like a neon billboard, followed by an image of the flight of stairs she would have to climb to get to the bathroom in the house. What exacerbated the situation is that she had never, ever liked using public restrooms. Ever! But, again, that was neither here nor there at that time. The choice was hers, and I wanted her to choose.

A few hours passed. Well, maybe not hours, but knowing that she had to use the bathroom, it sure felt like it.

"Mommy, do you have to use the bathroom now," I asked.

"No." This time, her voice was a little louder and a little more intense. This meant that she wanted me to stop asking her. Every time I asked her, she was reminded, Yes! I have to go, Janice!

We finally got home. "Mommy, you haven't used the bathroom since this morning. Don't you have to go?"

"Yes! And if we don't hurry up, its going to be down my leg!"

"Well, Mommy, why didn't you tell me? I knew you had to use the restroom. Why didn't you tell me?"

I was panicking. She was panicking. All the while, I was trying to get coordinated to do our "dance" up the stairs.

"Because of those stairs. I hate those stairs!" she said.

"Mommy, you need to start telling me. I don't want you to hold it like that. It's not good for you, okay?"

"Yeah."

"Okay, come on. Let's see if we can get up those stairs before it's too late. If we don't make it, hey, it's no big deal. But let's try. From now on, you have to tell me, okay?"

"Okay, I'm sorry."

"You don't have to say you're sorry, Mommy. I understand. Come on. I got you."

If you find yourself in this type of situation, try not to get so nervous that you make the stroke survivor feel bad. And in all honesty, remember Mommy NEVER liked to use public bathrooms, EVER! So, she was still the same person. Nothing had changed about that.

"Listen, we're going to have to concentrate, Mommy."

Mommy and I "danced" together to get up the first set of stairs leading to the front door. Together, in rhythm, I directed our moves like we were on a small ballroom floor with a little bit of muscle, gentle verbal cues and a lot of rhythm.

"Okay, step."

She planted her right leg firmly on the stairs. I pulled her up as she planted her left foot firmly on the stairs beside her right leg.

"And step . . . and step . . ." We take our time, always making sure each step is stable before the next one, but we kept moving. If Mommy thought too hard or deeply as she was physically moving, she'd get a little confused. So, we let it flow and kept dancing.

"Step . . . come on . . . let's get up these outside stairs first . . . hold it in, Mommy."

"Oh sh--, what have we gotten ourselves into, Janice?" We started to giggle.

We have been through this a million times. The laughing made us weaker. We had to stop laughing in order to move, and not just move, but move forward and up the stairs.

"Remember, the rule is no talking or laughing as we're going up the next flight of stairs," I reminded her.

"Okay, Janice. Let's go!"

We're in sync…we are ready. Up the stairs we continued to move.

"Okay . . . step . . . good . . . step . . . good . . ."

The whole way, we were both saying, "Sssshhh . . . sssshhhh," to remind ourselves to be quiet, concentrate and not laugh. Keep it moving, concentrate and don't be so loud . . . ssshhh . . . ssshhhh. Up the outside stairs, through the two front doors and up the final stairs to the top level.

Done! We danced all the way and finally made it to the bathroom, but it was a struggle. Bottom line is that we made it.

"That was close," Mommy said, smiling and sweating.

"Yeah, I know. But we did it, girlfriend!"

We smiled and wiped our foreheads as nature made its way into our lives and the commode.

Celebrate everything!

Riding the Rainbow

One thing to think about when you're in a situation like this as a caregiver is that sometimes it's not the fear you're dealing with when they say no. Sometimes they will say no because they don't want to bother you to ask for help. Other times it's just the way they are.

You may think your loved one has changed, and everything is the way it is because of a stroke. However, it may be a case of things remaining as they have always been and are still. It's good to remember that before they had the stroke, they never had to ask anyone to help them use the restroom, so it's very different for them now. Be patient and understanding if you can, because believe me, it's more difficult for them.

CHAPTER 9

The Buddy System

I haven't told you about the time my mom and one of her dearest friends, Ms. Rosetta Randall, thought they'd wrestle before going to the bathroom. Yep, that's right. WrestleMania, up close and personal!

While Mommy was in the hospital, Ms. Rosetta was helping her either onto the bed or trying to get her out of the bed. I couldn't tell from the position I found them in—on the floor with Mommy on top of Ms. Rosetta!

Anyway, as they later explained, Mommy and Ms. Rosetta were trying to go to the bathroom. There was some pulling as Ms. Rosetta tried to get Mommy off the bed. Mommy laughed and laughed and laughed, and then Ms. Rosetta started laughing too! They were laughing so hard, they could hardly speak, and that was the problem. As they were trying to get to the bathroom, they started laughing, lost their balance and footing. Then BAM! They fell onto the floor.

"Help! Help! Help!" Ms. Rosetta screamed, scared senseless.

That's when I came in.

At the sound of the bell signifying the end of the match, I'm happy to say, both were fine. It was a good laugh for us all. Ms. Rosetta made sure Mommy never hurt herself, even if that meant placing her body between Mommy and the floor. Ms. Rosetta was, and still is, one of the family. A precious gem.

Riding the Rainbow

Oh, wait! I must tell you the reason why Mommy even decided to walk to the bathroom in the first place instead of using one of those bedpans. The last time my father and I got Mommy's buttock onto and into the bedpan, we couldn't get it off! Her cute, little booty had slipped into the bedpan and was stuck. When we rolled her over, the bedpan went with her.

We laughed and laughed and laughed. We thought we'd never get that bed pan off that little hiney. So, from the pan—or Honey Pot, as they'd call it in the south—to the bathroom is progress. We call it a tiny-hiney bit of evolution!

CHAPTER 10

OOOOPPPPPPSSSSSSS

Depending on which side of the brain the stroke affected, you may find yourself in certain situations, be stuck in the middle of certain events, or have your back against the wall of certain events and all you can say is oooopppppssssss.

Like laughing at the wrong time.

One day, someone told Mommy that their dog had gone to pet heaven. Mommy kind of smiled and then burst out laughing. Of course, her reaction was inappropriate, but it wasn't her fault. Her brain was still having problems processing judgement, emotions, and subsequently, reactions. It was like an outside stimulus triggering something inside of her, visually or emotionally, but the message got jumbled up and crashed through the scar tissue in her brain.

Sometimes, by the time the brain gets the message and sends back a response—using pony express, of course—the reaction is not thoroughly thought out. These kinds of jumbled expressions happened so quickly that Mommy wouldn't have time to stop it or at least add a filter. The message took a right instead of a left, so the message sent back was from another region. Get it?

In situations like this, take care and keep it simple. Don't embarrass the stroke survivor. When Mommy responded to something inappropriately, I'd say something to the person like, "I'm sorry. She doesn't mean it. It's part of the healing and rehabilitation process."

Then I'd look at Mommy to bring her into the situation in a positive way and say, "Right, Mommy?"

"Right," she would quickly respond. "I apologize. I'm still healing."

Once we did that a few times, she took over. From then on, whenever

44

something like this happened again, she apologized and explained what happened and why in her own words. I loved when this happened because Mommy was reclaiming her voice. It also helped because I wasn't explaining or talking about Mommy, or for her, as if she wasn't present.

Ignoring someone or speaking for the survivor all the time can make the survivor feel ashamed. It can also increase the levels of guilt they may already be feeling. Speaking for a stroke survivor when they are present may be perceived as rude and demeaning, even if that is not your intention.

Using the power of social stories, I explained to Mommy that it wasn't her fault.

A social story is a simple story that describes a social situation and the appropriate way to act in that situation. I'd say with a smile, "Your brain got a little confused, and you've always been honest. Tell you what. Next time, take a moment, pause, edit, or revise the message in your head if you have to, then come up with the appropriate expression or response, okay? We can try that."

We talked about different scenarios and possible solutions until Mommy felt better.

Talking through different scenarios allows the stroke survivor to regain their personal agency and frees them from self-blame and guilt that can be counterproductive. Social stories benefit the stroke survivor in a myriad of ways, including:

Self-regulation and the management of one's emotions and behavior, which helps with building a new sense of resilience.

Improved social-emotional capacity. Talking about the emotions of others can help the stroke survivor better understand how their actions affect others.

A stroke takes up a lot of space and energy in the stroke survivor and their family/caregivers' lives. You must have an eye toward modifying your perspective and behavior. This helps you to adapt your approach towards a balanced mindset. Otherwise, the caregiving role can be quite overwhelming and stressful.

What I also found interesting were the residual effects of a stroke that can manifest in ways that are atypical of a person's normal behavior. For example, a person that was always confident and self-assured may now be insecure. Although there is a connection, the survivor, and sometimes caregivers, will see this new personality trait as a character flaw rather than a residual effect of the stroke. Not making this connection can often result in survivors getting the wrong type of attention, such as being called insecure or weak. Instead, we need to make sure we make the connection and remind and reassure the survivor that it is just the effects of the stroke. "Your brain is still healing," I used to tell Mommy.

As challenging as it may be at times to deal with this type of manifestation, we must treat survivors as if their personal agency is still intact. This means they can still speak up for themselves. That they still have a say in their behavior, if and whenever possible. The main thing to remember is that it is important the stroke survivor regain power and as much control as they can to move closer to their newly seeded hopes and dreams.

Mommy and I knew, as honest as she could be, she'd never say or do something to hurt someone's feelings, intentionally. This means she shouldn't be punished for something that was unintentional, and she had no control of due to medical reasons.

Speaking of good 'ole honesty, my mother became one of the most honest people in the world! Out loud! Verbally! That was one of the side effects from the stroke. Have you ever been in a situation when someone asks you something, but the response has the potential to blow up like a hundred sticks of dynamite?

"Hey, Vi! Do you like my dress?" asked a woman Mommy knew.

Mommy made a funny face and nervously looked at me. She signaled me through telepathy to help her and turned her lip up as she worked through the pausing and filtering steps I suggested to her before responding. I gave her an encouraging look and smiled.

She slowly turned to the woman and slowly opened her mouth. "Do you like it girlfriend?"

"Yes," the woman answered.

Mommy replied, "Great! That's all that matters, because if you like it, I love it!"

Whew, I thought. The woman walked away smiling.

I said with relief, "Great job, Mommy."

Mommy replied, "Girl, I was so nervous!"

Being as proud as punch, I said, "You did great!"

Mommy definitely came a long way, but as in life, other challenges were always waiting around the corner. One day a woman came toward us with a hairstyle that, if asked, I didn't even know if I could bend the truth about it!

Mommy quickly tried to turn her wheelchair around to speed away, and I was trying to play it cool and get out of the way, which made Mommy nervous. She ran into me and across my toe. Despite our best efforts, we got nowhere! And this woman was coming fast. Mommy was sweating and looking nervous.

"Don't look nervous, Mommy."

"Don't you look nervous, Janice."

My frazzled retort was, "I'm not looking nervous. You're looking nervous!"

Mommy exclaimed aloud, "Oh sh__!"

The woman with the curious hairstyle said, "Oh! There's Vi!" She walked even faster toward Mommy. As she got closer, I heard her say, "I've got to ask Vi how she likes my hair!"

And before we knew it . . .

"Hey, Vi!" she said excitedly.

Mommy said, "Hey, girlfriend!" She then said, quickly, "I wish I could talk, but Janice and I are late for an appointment, but I'll catch up with you a little later. Okay?" Mommy dropped that excuse, never letting go of the accelerator handle on her motorized wheelchair. Smooth.

"Okay then. Hi, Janice!" the woman yelled out as we zoom past her.

I responded as we moved forward. "Hi, Mrs. Blankety Blank. It's so great seeing you!" I pushed Mommy out the door, trying not to hit anyone.

That was a close call!

There can be other types of socially related effects of strokes to keep in mind, like over-confidence! Over-Confidence was in full effect at an event where Mommy was really dressed up. One of her friends said, "I love your dress, Vi. You look so pretty today."

Mommy responded, "I know."

And that was it. Another effect of the stroke.

Now this is great confidence, no doubt, but a little role playing, and the insertion here and there of a social story or two doesn't hurt, as they can make situations like this easier to manage.

Riding the Rainbow

So, Mommy and I role played. She played the woman, and I played her. Mommy said, "I like your dress. You look very pretty."

"I know!" I responded like Mommy had done and in the same tone.

This allowed Mommy to hear what it sounded like from the woman's perspective. Mommy burst out laughing.

"Oh my! I need to stop that, Janice."

I told her, "Now that we know better, we will do better."

I also reminded her that a lot of people in the world, including myself, could use practice with this. Not only did we get a good laugh out of it, but Mommy saw how her actions, verbal language, and tone, like any other human being, can affect someone else. Believe it or not, this was empowering for Mommy.

She existed. She was still normal, and this made her feel good.

CHAPTER 11

It is *too* Raining

Some stroke survivors kind of, sort of, accept the after-effects of the stroke. Many have choices and, to a large degree, their choice should be respected. But sometimes, they still believe that if they don't admit to something being wrong, then really and truly, nothing is wrong. It's called denial. It is also a case of wanting to control something directly related to their illness. A great example of this took place when Mommy was at the eye doctor.

Mommy was taking the eye test where you cover one eye and read a chart of letters with the other eye and then do the same thing in reverse. I happened to be sitting beside Mommy and saw her cheat! When the eye doctor turned to the chart to make sure Mommy was reading the letters correctly, she'd move the little paddle over ever so slightly to read with both eyes! When the doctor turned to her, she quickly covered one eye.

When I saw Mommy cheating, I thought to myself, heck, they won't let her drive, so what's it hurting?

Another time, I noticed that Mommy had shortness of breath. I walked into her room and asked, "Mommy, are you okay? Are you breathing okay?"

"Yes, I'm fine." This was always her response.

I knew I'd have to deal with these issues eventually. For a short time, I kept in mind that in our family, as in a lot of families who were Christian-focused or optimistic, we believed that if one did not speak about a topic, it didn't exist. The mindset was: claim nothing and it won't claim you.

We didn't speak of things we didn't want to manifest. The reality is things do exist and sometimes we must claim certain things before they claim us. It's a matter of balance.

One day, I noticed Mommy's left arm move up involuntarily. She'd quickly grabbed it and pulled it back down to her body.

I said, "Hey, Mommy. What was that?"

Mommy replied with an air of impatience, and I could see that she was bothered. "Nothing. Can I have some privacy please?"

Dealing with what I call the "visibly invisible" can be tricky. The first thing to remember is, if you think it's a challenge watching this, think of how the stroke survivor feels. It's happening to them directly and personally. So, step outside of the situation, keep calm and talk with the survivor. Let them know in a subtle way that you noticed also, but it's okay. Assure them that everything is going to be okay.

We're on top of it, together.

You are not alone; I got you.

Remember what I said about adaptation and modification? This is how it happened for us. Now, as I walk you through this process, the same type of ordeal you may have to address, I want you to keep in mind that some things can and will become better. There is a mental, emotional, psychological and spiritual tone that can be used in your approach and the handling of the somewhat awkward situation. I found that staying positive is a great way to approach most things. Do what you can, within reason, to make the stroke survivor feel as comfortable as possible and, by all means, play to your strong suit. For me, it was leading with a blend of compassion, listening, encouragement and a sense of humor.

Despite her arm having a mind of its own (doctors call it an alien hand), I assured Mommy that everything was going to be okay. The next time her arm acted up, I laughed and yelled like I discovered gold!

I thought about the involuntary arm motions. "Your left arm was your dominant arm, Mommy, and I'm sure it wants to help too."

Her arm was still there like she was, and from that point on, we worked on controlling her left arm a little more each day. The upside was that Mommy's brain was working. It was just still healing. Her eyes saw a pocket, and her brain said, "Hey! There's a pocket! It must be yours! Put your hand into the pocket."

So, Mommy put her hand into the pocket. Any pocket! It didn't have to be hers.

"We need to take that arm to Vegas! No one will ever suspect a pickpocket to be a woman in a wheelchair. We're going to be rich!" I said.

We both laughed. Of course, we were kidding, but it's one of those things.

Eventually, after practice, this involuntary arm phenomenon went away.

The next time we went to the eye doctor, Mommy, of course, cheated again. This time, I whispered into her ear, "I know you're cheating, and I won't tell this time, but you owe me five dollars."

That got a laugh.

I prepared Mommy for the next appointment by telling her, "There will be no cheating this time, Mommy. We want to know what's going on and how we can improve."

Mommy smirked and looked at me as the party spoiler. When she took her third vision test, she didn't cheat and only missed a few letters.

"Did I pass, doctor?" Mommy asked.

"You sure did," he said.

Mommy smiled really big and stuck her tongue out at me.

I praised Mommy for doing her very best. "Great job, Mommy! You only missed a few of them. Now we can move onto the next process."

I could tell she was proud instead of nervous.

Then it was time for me to revisit the breathing problem. I walked into her room. "Mommy, I see you're having problems breathing again. What do you think is wrong?"

Taking a proactive approach, I added, "I'm in this with you."

She replied, "I don't know. I think it's my allergies or maybe the way I'm lying down."

I nodded. "Okay. Why don't we try sitting in the chair for a few minutes? Maybe that will help."

This approach immediately let her know that I knew something was going on, so she didn't have to lie or avoid talking about it. As a caregiver or loved one, the key is to embrace the problem and then do something about it—together.

I always wanted Mommy to feel free to talk with me so that neither she nor I would be blindsided by anything. This takes purposeful nurturing, but if you do this and you're sincere, before you know it, you'll gain traction and they'll gain confidence. You may learn all the little things that are wrong and have been wrong for some time, which is invaluable when it comes to getting the survivor the correct treatment as they recover.

Riding the Rainbow

Mommy said, "Yeah, girl, my hip was hurting a little yesterday, and my arm was stiff. I'm trying to wiggle my toes, but they don't work all the time. I think my eyesight is clearing up, and I'm glad I can hear better now that we got that wax out. I thought something was really wrong with me."

Good Lord! All of that? I said to myself. We both giggled, smiled and reconnected.

Once everything is out on the table, you'll witness the stroke survivor gaining courage, self-empowerment and acceptance in a healthy way— with transparency and honesty. You're going to hear everything, but that's okay. This process takes some of the shame, embarrassment and worry away.

CHAPTER 12

Losing Track of Time

Depending on which side of the brain the stroke affected, there can be temporal issues and timing challenges. There was one rehabilitation exercise that Mommy always dreaded. She had to stand on her own or with the help of a walker for a specific duration of time.

Before her time was up, she'd call out, "Janice, can you please help me sit down? I've been standing here for almost an hour."

I looked at the clock. Two minutes had passed.

"I'm coming. Give me five minutes," I responded, trying to get her to reach the time goal.

Earlier that day, Mommy had a lot on her mind, but when I asked her what was wrong, she had refused to talk about it.

Mommy said, "I'm ready to talk now." I'm sure she was trying to get out of the rest of her standing exercise.

"Okay, Mommy, give me five," still trying to get her to her timing goal.

Now, she was really upset, because she had to either keep standing or learn to sit down on her own. That was the goal of the exercise, and it made her nervous.

Mommy was miffed. "It's already been five times five times five times five!"

I heard the nervousness and fear in her voice, so I helped her sit on the side of the bed.

Scenarios like this happened often at the beginning of her recovery. By the time Daddy, my sister, my brother Clifton and other helpers worked with Mommy, she had become more independent. When Mommy got tired of waiting on other people to help her, she helped herself to a seat whenever she wanted.

But her ability to stand on her own for lengths of time increased as well!

Riding the Rainbow

There were times when Mommy was like this because she really missed me being around her physically. When Daddy was working, she and I were together from about seven in the morning until the evening. I kept her company whenever I could, until she was okay sitting by herself, which eventually happened.

However, there were days when she wasn't as confident and times when she was deep in thought about how her life had changed since the stroke. She couldn't just get up, walk out to the car and go visit friends or her children by herself. She couldn't go back to work. During these times, Mommy felt lonely. Fortunately, those times didn't last for long.

The main thing to remember as a caregiver/loved one is when you feel, see, or hear something that catches your attention, pay attention. Trust your instincts and know that something is going on. It could be something serious or something benign like just wanting to have a conversation.

Mommy might say to me, "Did I tell you what Daddy and I had to eat for dinner yesterday?"

You must have patience and empathy. The outcome can be delightful. Just repeat the mantra: Patience. Patience. Patience.

CHAPTER 13

The Real You: When It Comes Blurting Out

After a stroke, you may notice that the survivor may seem more nervous than usual. The nervousness may be a reaction to the level of noise in the room, too many people around or plain anxiety. As a result, their true feelings may come blurting out. Don't take things personally. They're frustrated.

One day, Mommy and I went to the hair salon as we did each Thursday, every week. We got out of the car and made it to the front door before the owner stopped us and asked us to use the back entrance because it was closer to where Mommy would first get her hair washed. She hated having to turn around in front of people, and it showed. She was visibly upset, but she didn't say anything until she turned around to head back to the car. She was not pleased with me, and I could tell.

"I wish we would have just gone ahead in, Janice!" Mommy said.

To minimize any fallout, I replied, "Okay, Mommy, but we're here in the car now, so let's go to the back like he wants us to do."

She was very upset with me. We drove around to the back and entered the salon, and the frustration continued. Now, Mommy had to walk again, and she didn't want any more eyes on her. She was nervous about how she would look when she walked or turned around. She didn't want to be embarrassed. Unfortunately, things escalated.

For the first time, getting Mommy into the salon chair itself became a problem, because she was not only nervous, but she was also irritated. She wanted to sit down NOW! As I was doing the usual dance with her to make sure she sat in the chair safely, she kept trying to hastily sit down, but I wouldn't let her. She was too far away from the actual seat.

I called out, "Two more steps, Mommy."

Because she was nervous, her steps were small and unsure. I had to say it again. "Two more steps, Mommy."

She pulled back from me in haste. Finally, she got so frustrated she threw herself into the chair. Luckily, she made it and didn't hurt herself. She didn't like all the attention she got from the other patrons in the salon. They were merely concerned about her safety. I was nervous and upset, which only made Mommy even more upset.

I reminded her, "Mommy, you shouldn't do that. We've been practicing and practicing, and you could have hurt yourself."

She said, "Don't yell at me!"

"I'm not yelling at you, Mommy. I'm just saying . . ."

Again, Mommy frowned. "Don't yell at me!"

I felt awful because she was mad at me. In the moment, I raised my voice because I was afraid, nervous and probably a little frustrated.

"I'm sorry, Mommy. I want you to be more careful, okay?"

Mommy responded, "I don't like when you yell at me."

"Okay, I'm sorry. But I wasn't yelling. I was speaking a little louder than usual because I was nervous, and my throat muscles tightened up a little bit, okay?"

I was trying to explain my actions, which was both good and bad. Being transparent was good, because Mommy needed to know what was happening and that my feelings mattered as well. Most caregivers forget that they are human too and have emotions that need to be considered from time to time, depending on the situation. It was also bad because while all of this was happening, I hadn't considered that Mommy's hearing may have been a little sensitive, that her pride was involved or even that she felt confident enough that we didn't have to come in through the back.

I should have watched my tone and volume. I should have realized that she might be embarrassed. The matter was compounded because I was irritated too. While I was always checking up on Mommy, I felt that sometimes someone needed to check on me too.

I was always focused on keeping Mommy safe, and I couldn't figure out why Mommy would yell at me.

Riding the Rainbow

After we made it through the salon appointment, we went home and to our usual place: the bathroom, or what everyone in my family calls, The Throne. I hugged Mommy as she sat on the throne.

"I'm sorry. I'm sorry, okay? Do you forgive me?" I asked her. "I'm sorry, okay?" I kissed her right cheek.

She smiled big and wide, totally content. "Yes, okay."

"Good." I let out a sigh of relief, finally exhaling for the day.

"I'm sorry too," Mommy said.

I knew Mommy was tired too.

"It's okay. I understand, Mommy. We were emotionally sensitive today, but we meant well."

Thinking that Mommy and I had settled that issue, I walked out of the bathroom and down the hall when I heard Mommy say under her breath, "Turd!"

I quickly turned around, ran into the bathroom like I was going to leap on the top of her head. We both laughed.

Momma said there'd be days like this. Days of just being human. We are all in this together and whenever you can, try to find peace, make peace and say that you're sorry.

CHAPTER 14

Your Biggest Fan: Manipulation Begs Attention

Picture this: Mommy sitting on the side of her bed with a ceiling fan twirling above her.

Mommy yelled, "Janice, I'm hot!"

I walked down the hall and turned the ceiling fan to level one. I left the room.

Mommy yelled again, "I'm still hot!"

I stopped, sighed, walked back to the room and switched the fan to level two. I walked out, but before I could get down the hall, Mommy shouted, "Lord, I'm still hot!"

I turned around and turned the fan on full blast with a devious look on my face.

Mommy's napkin on the lunch tray took flight, flying around the room like a scene out of *The Wizard of Oz*. The drapes swished, and her hair blew in the ceiling fan breeze.

"There! How's that?" I asked her. I walked out of the room and down the hall.

Mommy shouted, "I'm cold! I'm cold!"

I walked back to the room and shut the fan completely off.

In a frustrated tone, I asked, "There! Happy"?

Not to be out done, Mommy said, "That's perfect."

I thought, *what kind of game is Mommy playing today?* I walked out of the room and down the hall. Then very softly, I heard those beautiful words, "Ole turd."

I quickly ran back to the room and jumped on the bed, wrapping my arms lightly around her entire body and growled. We laughed.

"What in the world is wrong with you, Mommy?" I asked.

She told me, "I needed some attention."

"Really? I'll give you some attention!" I wrapped my hands around her neck, playfully choking her.

Mommy laughed uncontrollably. She was ticklish around the neck.

"Next time, just tell me."

Gleefully, she said, "Okay."

Riding the Rainbow

Everyone in my family could be a brat from time to time. This was normal for us. Mommy was funny and playful, and I was like her. The play and bantering were what we did in our household.

Getting through life's hard times is so much easier if there is an infinite source of humor. For our family, humor was crucial, especially in situations where feelings could be hurt. If humor doesn't work, you can look at these challenges as motivation to get up and do something for yourself–a win-win situation!

CHAPTER 15

It's Not Easy Being Me

It's not easy being a stroke survivor. For a lot of big and small reasons. We all get frustrated in life, so as a caregiver, expect moments of real frustration from the survivor from time to time. As you have already learned, there may be moments of short tempers and impatience, even times when things can become a little physical. Try to remember to be understanding, patient, have a sense of humor and be quick to duck!

Mommy was sitting in her wheelchair in front of Daddy, who was standing up in front of her. She kept moving her head from the left to the right like she was dodging something we couldn't see. Then I saw it!

Daddy had put on one of his favorite shirts, but it was a little tight around the mid-section. It looked like a button was going to pop right off and hit Mommy square in the eye!

"Oh gosh! It's going to poke my eye out," Mommy yelled.

We laughed and laughed, and of course, Daddy changed his shirt.

Then there were times when things weren't as funny. One time, Mommy was tired and irritable, and I was trying to get her in the car. She just stood there. She didn't want to do anything but be defiant.

"Mommy, can we get in the car?"

She said nothing.

"Are we just going to stand here and chill?"

Again, Mommy said nothing.

She finally allowed me to help her sit down in the car, but then she refused to pull her legs in.

Exercising patience and self-empowerment, I said, "Okay, Mommy, go ahead and get your legs in the car."

Mommy was resistant to say the least. "No. Stop! Leave me alone."

"Mommy, I'm trying to help you." I gently tried to get her legs into the car. We lightly tussled a bit. To add to the tussling, I was hot—not attitude-wise, but physically hot.

The sun beamed on the left side of my face as I was doing all of this. I mean, the sun was beating down on top of us! Mommy pushed me as I worked to get her legs into the car. WHAM! I took a right hook to the ole kisser!

Don't worry; it was a very light right hook. I looked at Mommy. She looked at me.

"I'm goin getcha!" I said.

We began to laugh. It was just one of those moments.

Riding the Rainbow

Mommy was having a hard moment and a hard day. She was absolutely, positively over all of it! She was over therapy, exercising, lack of freedom and independence. You name it. She was being defiant because she could.

It was good that she was tired of being told what to do. She was tired of dealing with the residual effects from the stroke, day in and day out. She was mad that it happened to her, and she always had to find a new way of doing things. How to walk, talk, sleep and drive. Add to that, she was always trying to stay positive. I'm sure it was hard. Putting a positive slant on our situation, Mommy's defiant attitude meant that she wanted to do better. That was wonderful!

Sometimes—many times—it doesn't seem fair to the stroke survivor or the caregiver(s) to have to go through this. It isn't. But, at the same time, having or not having a stroke isn't about fairness. It's about change—something that can happen to anyone at any time.

Stay positive and proactive. If you find yourself frustrated and the person you are caring for is becoming increasingly defiant or ill-tempered, continue to do what you can, when you can, and however you can. It's a good idea for caregivers to learn how to forgive, talk about it, forget about it, move on, and for goodness sake, duck!

CHAPTER 16

The Biting Effect

Other than the story about Daddy's shirt button, I never gave much thought to how height could play an important role in nervousness and have such a biting effect.

Once, early in the healing process, Mommy and I were making our way up the stairs. She was nervous, so it was a bit challenging, step by step. Mommy was afraid she was going to fall backward, or I was going to lose my grip on her. Her arms and legs didn't always respond when and how she wanted. She wasn't confident.

I always told Mommy, when fear is at its highest, do whatever you have to do to stay safe. If you think you're about to fall, grab what you can, with what you can to stay safe.

Boy oh boy, did she ever take that advice seriously and literally! Painfully so!

As we walked up the stairs one leg and foot at a time, Mommy repeated, "I'm scared. I'm scared."

To keep her calm, I said, "It's okay, Mommy. I got you."

Despite my efforts, she wasn't convinced. "Janice, I'm scared."

She was stressed out, so I tried to offer encouragement. "Stay calm. I got you, okay?"

It didn't seem to ease her anxiety. "I'm going to fall!"

Her apprehension kicked in, and there was no way I could convince her that she wasn't going to fall.

All I could do was stay the course and keep us moving. Again, trying to assure her that she was safe and sound, I said, "No, you're not, Mommy. Please calm dowwwwwwnnnnnnn."

No matter what I said, she felt that she was going to fall. So, she did exactly what I had always told her to do in a situation such as that–she reached out with whatever she could and grabbed onto the first thing she could to stop herself from falling.

Since I had both of Mommy's arms, she used the only thing she could—her teeth! She bit down tightly on my shirt, which meant loosely, innocently, but painfully, had a hold of the tiniest bit of something else without knowing it! Ouch!

Sweating, painfully, slowly, I said, "It's okay, Mommy. I got you. Please let go now. Loosen up. Let it go, Mommy. Let it go!"

As I was pleading with Mommy to release me, she was laughing and giggling uncontrollably, which meant that she couldn't let go. She was still afraid of falling, and her brain needed her to stop one thing before she could do another. I'm sure she was going for the shirt, but when you're panicked, you do the best that you can. After a few seconds that felt like a lifetime of me pulling away from Mommy, she stopped laughing, and I was finally free!

Mommy said, "Sorry, baby. I was afraid I was going to fall. I was so nervous."

Using the best line of humor I could muster, I told her, "That's okay, Mommy. I understand. You did the best you could. They're big, and they're there for the grabbing or biting. I just didn't have you in mind doing it!"

We both let out a long laugh!

"If that happens again, do you think you could come up with another solution that's a little less painful?"

We laughed so hard and long, I thought we were going to have to go through the entire process again, because we were still on the stairs.

"Yes, we could work on it," Mommy said, still laughing.

All I could say was, "Great. Thanks so much. Now let's go, so that I can get me some ice."

It's too funny the things we go through and come through, right?

Riding the Rainbow

The main thing to remember or the main thing I remember from this situation is that I was really happy Mommy did exactly what I told her to do whenever she felt unsafe. She took action and saved herself! That was awesome! She still had some fight in her, and I could not have been prouder.

Chapter 17

And Another Thing

Healing by empowerment is when you learn how to get through various situations by using your strengths, addressing your weaknesses, and taking responsibility. That's empowerment! This can be challenging for survivors because they don't have the same control they used to have over their lives and bodies. This can also mean that, suddenly, the stroke survivors need to control something, anything or someone. I think it's only human nature.

For example, one day Mommy looked at the clock Daddy placed by her bed and said, "I'm going to sleep now, Janice."

"Okay, nappy nap," I responded. Instead of me or Daddy looking at the clock and telling Mommy that it was time for her to nap according to schedule, she took it upon herself to decide when she was going to sleep. Not me, not Daddy or even the clock.

After I finished my chores and the meals were cooked, Mommy and I had to compromise on what we were going to watch on television. I say compromise, but my mom usually won. However, when she was sleeping, the world and the universe of television was all mine! All mine, I say!

I had a strategy. I sat quietly and watched her eyelids slowly begin to close. *Yes, Mommy, go to sleepy sleep. Hee hee hee.*

When she was finally sleeping, I cautiously and slowly leaned over to grab the television remote control from her sleeping hand.

With her eyes still closed, Mommy said, "Janice, leave my remote control alone."

Darn!

I couldn't watch television in another room because she wanted my company, and I loved being around her. At least while she napped, I should be able to watch something on TV I selected.

I waited a little while longer. Good. She went into a deeper sleep; I heard her quietly purring. I went for the TV remote again. *Yes! I got it!*

I had the remote control in the palm of my hand. Suddenly, Mommy's hand shot out, and her fingernails closed on my hand! *Yikes! Stopped again!*

Not to be outfoxed, I went for plan C. I acted as if I was quietly leaving to use the ladies' room. When I knew she was sleeping, I snuck back into the room and looked for the remote. But I couldn't find it. It wasn't in her hand or near her body. *Where could it be?*

It wasn't under her face, where she would sometimes leave it, and wake up with remote button imprints on her face. I looked around the bed. The remote was not on the dresser and not on the floor. Darn! I had no luck in finding it, so I decided to go to sleep too.

A little while later, I woke up to the sound of someone surfing the channels. Mommy was flipping through the channels at record speed.

"Hey, Mommy! Where was the remote control? I couldn't find it anywhere."

With a healthy dose of momma-bear attitude and self-agency, she replied, "I know. I knew you were coming after my remote control, so, I put it under my pillow and slept on it."

Dope!

That was a game we played all the time—hide the remote. I loved it and so did she. This game of hide and seek also helped to keep her brain active.

Having some sense of power makes us feel safe, more secure. I started wondering what more I could do to make sure Mommy still felt powerful and not helpless. So, the Navy Seal training began, and I was the instructor. First lesson: how to defend yourself.

"Mommy, I don't want you to be a helpless victim. If you need to fight, I want you to fight. With all that you have! Now don't be afraid. You won't hurt me."

I pushed her while she was sitting on the bed. "Fight me back! Defend yourself! Hit me with your right fist!"

Pow! She hit me!

"Hit me with your left."

Pow! She hit me!

"Yeah, yeah, yeah. Good, Mommy!"

And there she was. There was Mommy again, ready to protect and fight.

"I'll scratch your eyes out! I'll kick you! Don't push me! I'll hit you with this book! I'll crack your head with this phone," she started yelling. She really got into it.

"Whoa, Mommy! Slow down. I think you got it. Let's move on." I wanted to keep the momentum.

"Mommy, what if something happens to me? What would you do?"

"I guess you're out of luck," she said.

"Come on, Mommy. I'm serious. I want you to yell 9-1-1."

Mommy quietly said, "9 1 1."

"Mommy, no one can hear that!" I imitated her whispering. "Really yell it, Mommy! 9-1-1! I need help! Yell for help! 9-1-1!"

"9-1-1," she said with a little more enthusiasm.

"Better! Now say it louder!"

"9-1-1!"

"Better, louder!"

"Help! Help me! 9-1-1!"

"Better, louder!"

"Help! Help me! 9-1-1!"

"Better, louder!"

"9-1-1," Mommy shouted. "Help me, somebody! My daughter has lost her mind, and she won't leave me alone! 9-1-1! 9-1-1!"

We laughed hysterically! Mommy was so funny.

"Okay, cool. So, I don't have to worry about you, right?"

"Right. Now leave me alone. I'm watching TV."

"Okay, but first, what's my phone number?"

Mommy was confident and sure of herself. "Six-six-six."

She laughed out loud.

I didn't give up. "Mommy, that's not funny. What's my phone number?"

In a frustrated tone, she gave it a shot. "Oh sssshhhh . . . five five five . . . nine two . . . I don't know."

Always being proactive, I responded, "Okay. I'm going to ask Daddy to add my phone number to this list you have here, and I want you to memorize it, okay?"

"Yes, Janice. Sure." She smirked, like *yeah right*. "Now can I watch

TV?"

"Yep, right after you repeat after me. Five five five."

"Five five five."

"Nine two six five."

"Nine two six five."

"Now you say it."

"Five five five . . . nine two six five."

"Again."

"Five five five . . . nine two six five."

"Good."

Later that evening, when I was at my home, I called her.

Mommy answered, "Hello?"

"What's up, shortay?"

"Hey, girlfriend."

"Hey, Mommy!"

"Yeah?" I could tell by her tone that she knew something was up.

"Let's practice. I need help. Call me."

Mommy started to laugh. "Janice, you're a fool!"

"Call me, Mommy. I'm hanging up now, so don't forget. Call me."

I hung up and waited . . . and waited . . . and waited.

I called Mommy back.

She answered the phone. "Hello?"

"Mommy! Why didn't you call me back?"

"Because I didn't want to."

"Mommy, it's an exercise. Do you want me to leave you alone?"

"Yes," she declared.

"Are you sure?"

True to form, Mommy sarcastically said, "Positive."

"Then when I hang up, call me back. Okay?"

She said, "Anything to get you to leave me alone!"

I hung up once again and waited.

Ring ring.

I answered, "Hello, Collins' residence."

"Can I watch TV now?" she asked.

"Yay, Mommy, you did it."

I smiled, so proud of her.

Riding the Rainbow

It's hard for parents to take direction from their children when they have been in charge their whole lives. All that pushing and pulling resulted in Mommy calling me every day. I felt good that she was checking on me and that she could call for help. I also enjoyed her calling me *just to chat*. I say just to chat because it's good to remember not to center your whole life or their whole life around the stroke. I encourage you to talk to talk. Laugh to laugh and live in the present. Take a break from the medical stuff and get back to a sense of normalcy whenever possible. It makes handling things a lot easier. Remember, healing from the stroke as a caregiver can be a part of your life, but it doesn't have to be your life.

I also want to mention that sleeping can be challenging for those who have survived a stroke. They can be anxious going to sleep, not knowing if they will be better or worse when they wake up. Will a miracle happen, or was it all just a dream? The world around them and their home suddenly seems excessively quiet. This quietness can give them time and space to think about their problems, illnesses, and how they are going to make it through the day. The same feelings that many of us have felt and feel. So, having the television on or music playing quietly in the background or having someone around when they're sleeping can really help stabilize the survivors' nerves.

Just knowing that someone is there watching over them while they sleep can bring them comfort, because they feel that if something happens to them in the middle of their nap, someone is there to take care of them. It's nice to know that someone is there.

CHAPTER 18

Use It or Lose It

One thing you must be consistent with until it becomes a habit is getting the stroke survivor to use whatever side of the body that the stroke affected. Continue to make them use the weaker side of the body to establish balance. They must use it, so they don't lose it.

The body is one big machine. When there is a weak side, another player on the team will take over and try to make up for it. This is a good thing, but it's only supposed to be temporary. For instance, if the left leg is the weak leg, survivors will work more and harder on the right side, which, yes, keeps them moving and that's a good thing.

However, if they continue to only use the strong side, that's the only side that will get stronger. The weaker side will continue to weaken every day, and the body will become unbalanced. Because of this, Mommy and our family believed in a consistent approach to therapy. We were wholeheartedly committed to physical therapy, inside and outside of the home. Staying physical was part of our regular routine.

When in the role as caregiver, try to match the physical activity with the capacity of the person you are caring for. There are endless options you can suggest to the stroke survivor: lifting weights, riding a stationary bike, swimming, or moving their legs and arms while sitting or lying down.

The most common and effective activity you can get the survivor to do, if they are able, is walking. No matter the activity, keep the body moving because experts and doctors can't predict what will happen in each case. Prognoses vary so they must take it on a case-by-case basis and so should you. Even if you must help your loved one move their body while they are in bed or sitting in a chair, keep that body alive and kicking!

Riding the Rainbow

The potential and predictions for partial or full recovery is as deep and as wide as the universe. There's no telling what the stroke survivor can accomplish. And it feels good to keep trying, for both the survivor and the caregiver. Don't give up and don't give in. Keep at it and, most importantly, keep moving. You never know.

Mommy went from not being able to use her left arm and leg for quite some time to getting full movement with the help of the physical therapists, Daddy, my sister Sharon (who used to be an RN), myself, other immediate and extended family members, and friends. That story is coming up soon. I encourage you to enjoy and celebrate the journey.

CHAPTER 19

It's All in the Head

I advise to not only work to strengthen the physically weaker side of the body, but also the weaker side of the brain. Routines and repetition are the best teachers. For example, one activity that many stroke survivors can do is answer the phone in their own home. Trust me when I say, practice makes perfect.

Mommy answered the house phone one day, and as the person on the other end was speaking, she looked at the base and hung up the phone. Like the Vegas Alien Arm analogy, when she saw the base of the landline phone, her brain told her that the phone handset should be on the base. So, she put the receiver down on the phone base without cognitive thinking. It was visual thinking. No goodbye. No thank you for calling. No see you later. Just click.

The phone rung another day. This time, I whispered to her, "Waaaiiiitttt."

Mommy was listening to the person talking on the other end of the phone, but every time she looked at the base, I could tell she was eager to hang up. Her brain was telling her the next logical step—visually. Forget the conversation; you see the phone base for the receiver, hang up! So, she again hung up right in the middle of the person talking.

I always thought it was sooooo funny to watch! I can only imagine what the person on the other end was thinking. Mommy couldn't help it.

It was time to do some retraining. I proceeded with a tutorial and social story to nurture the new phone protocol. "Mommy, when the phone rings, let them say something, listen to what they are saying, then wait for a moment of silence, then you say something, then wait for them to respond. Until they say goodbye, stay present with the conversation, listen and concentrate. When they say goodbye and *after* you say goodbye, then hang up. Try that next time."

Mommy acknowledged what I said with a heart okay.

She could follow directions that were simple and direct while her brain was healing and redesigning itself with new inroads of communication. I didn't talk down to her. I used a positive and proactive style, always with an eye toward affirming and encouraging her.

Another opportunity presented itself for us to practice the new telephone protocol. The phone rang.

"Hello," she answered.

The caller said, "Hey, there! I was wondering if you would be interested in one million free minutes of long distance?"

Mommy quickly replied, "No thank you."

The caller responded in kind, "Okay, thank you, ma'am."

Mommy used her new skills adeptly, telling the caller, "Bye. Have a nice day."

Then, like a well-oiled machine, I heard a click. She hung up the phone. The social stories and tutorials were engaged, and Mommy applied what we had practiced. I was so happy and proud in that moment. "Yay! You did a great job!"

To further strengthen the new phone protocol, a friend of mine agreed to help me out with this activity. Now beware, once the As and Bs are in place, the stroke survivor may feel a little more comfortable, like themselves again, which means that their personality may also come back full tilt.

The phone practice resumed. The phone rang. The caller said, "Hello ma'am. Would you be interested in two million free minutes for long distance?"

Mommy promptly replied, "Not interested." Click.

And that response was the real thing, processed with personality. She was never a big fan of spam sales calls. Kudos to you, Mommy.

Oh yeah, one more thing. When the survivor starts doing their own thing on the phone, keep an ear out to make sure they don't sell the house or buy a new one! But remember that if they do something like this, they didn't mean it.

There were other practices that were helpful. Mommy always washed and folded our clothes. When she had her stroke, I started doing this chore. I wasn't the best at this so clothes started shrinking and coming out in different colors. I'm so glad Daddy never got mad at suddenly wearing pink socks, underwear and tee-shirts, that used to be white. This was a wonderful opportunity for Mommy to step in. "Mommy, Daddy is going to be so mad at me! I turned his socks pink again! And look at this tee-shirt! It looks like a 5-year olds'!" Mommy started to laugh loud and hard.

"Please help me. With all of the different colors, I get confused."

"Okay, Janice, I'll help you. You're so pitiful," she says.

"Thanks so much Mommy! Now, tell me what to do."

From that point on, Mommy was not only in charge of separating and helping me with the wash, she also helped me with the folding. I would give her the towels and face towels to fold so that she could work both sides of her brain and both arms. She was really helping me and I wanted her to know how much I appreciated it. "I still have to cook dinner. Thank you so much for your help Mommy." She really enjoyed taking care of the same household chores again. We worked great as a team and it was another way for us to bond and give Mommy purpose! That is so important in anyone's life.

There will be moments when the stroke survivor will have a short attention span or lose things they know they had. It's not all in their head. One day, Mommy was changing the channels every three seconds. We all can be a little like this from time to time, can't we? We can't decide what to watch on the TV.

I said, "Mommy, I'm not watching this movie with you if you're going to keep changing the channels every five seconds."

Being my mom, she either said, "Okay, I won't," and kept on flipping the channels, or she said, "Then get out!" and laughed.

Either way, it was a normal response, and that's where we're heading—the new normal that returns to the old normal.

Other times, she'd change the subject matter right in the middle of a conversation you're having. When things like this happened, the first thing I did was smile. She didn't mean it, remember? Or did she? During one of our drives, we were having a conversation. "Mommy, I saw Mama Dip on TV today and---"

"I want to go to the mall today to pick out a yellow dress," she interrupted.

I thought, Whoa... "Hello? Can I please finish my story?"

Without missing a beat, she said, "Hurry up!" and smirked.

We both laughed, and I continued to tell my boring story that we could have lived without hearing, and Mommy patiently listened. At least I think she was listening. I finished my story.

She said, "Whew! Is it my turn to talk now?"

I laughed. "Sure, go ahead, Mommy."

"Thank you!" We both laughed as she told her story.

When my mother had a short attention span in public with someone else, I'd gently touch her on the leg or lightly on the hand and smile, signaling to her to wait a moment, stay present and listen. I didn't want to embarrass her.

This strategy was one we had talked about in advance of our regular outings. Before an outing, Mommy and I had a conversation about this technique in the car. We talked about how we were going to engage in social etiquette and what she wanted to do and not do in public. More importantly, we talked about what she felt comfortable doing. With the social stories and a plan of action, we were ready for the next situation.

Speaking of short attention span, there's also the case of lost and found. Here and there, Mommy lost things. This can be a normal occurrence after having a stroke. One afternoon, I heard her fussing a bit.

"I can't find my comb and I had it!" Mommy sounded a bit concerned. She always liked to look nice. I'm sure she was thinking about my father was coming home soon and wanting to look her best.

I encouraged and calmed her down. "Mommy, look around really good, because unless you went running down the hall and hid it, it's still in this room somewhere. Look around really good now."

She was frustrated and repeated what was now a mantra. "I had it. I know I did."

"Don't get frustrated. Let's think about it. You know you had it right?"

Mommy replied, "Right."

I slowly took her back through her time in the room. "Where's the one place you need to pay extra special attention to?"

She looked to her weak side—her left side—and there it was. Her comb. She smiled. "I got it!"

She stuck her tongue out at me and all was right with the world.

Riding the Rainbow

Lesson learned. Critical thinking is active. Mommy helped herself, achieved a goal by herself and life went on. Isn't life good?

CHAPTER 20

Everyone Do-si-do!

Like a good ole square dance or line dance, everyone in the family can and should participate in the care and nurturing of the stroke survivor. Let's say you don't want to participate, or you don't know how. Everyone, including the survivor, will notice your absence, and the dynamics in the family will be affected.

On the other hand, if you do decide to participate, that will also be noticed. Keep it simple. Bring what you already do best to the table. If you don't have anything that you do well, come to the table anyway and collaborate with everyone. Your energy and company will be greatly appreciated. It's about a beautiful, encouraging and positive unified front to help tackle each day, each accomplishment and challenge with and for the survivor.

My brother Clifton lifted weights with my mother. My brothers Ronald and Donald laughed and cracked jokes with Mommy.

"Mommy, which twin am I?" Ronald asked, as Donald sang in the background.

My brother Michael is an artist, and he showed Mommy how to write her name by using her visual imagination and other forms of drawing and writing.

Aunt Jackey and Aunt Delores called to share a good laugh or the latest happenings in the family. Sharon, my sister, taught Mommy how to walk without a cane and how to go over her medications. Miss Rosetta and other family friends kept Mommy company and made her laugh. Miss Rosetta also cooked delicious meals like homemade chicken and dumplings!

And Daddy was Daddy—giving Mommy what none of us could give her . . . those kisses and love essential between a husband and wife. "I love you, baby," Daddy said often.

"Hey, baby." She was forever flirting, telling Daddy, "You smell so good, and you look good too! Come here and let me kiss you."

Mommy always found time to flirt with Daddy. All of this is part of the healing, repair and loving process of being partners. Even if the survivor and their partner didn't do positive things before the stroke, there are always new beginnings. Encourage them to kiss, kiss, kiss. I'll talk more about romance and Daddy in a later chapter.

Riding the Rainbow

Pay attention, caregivers. Everyone will play a part in the recovery process one way or another, good or bad, positive, or negative. It's up to each of you what role you will play and the tone of this role. I know you'll try hard and make the right decision or the best decision that you can make. Just try to stay open and positive.

CHAPTER 21

Keep Moving

No matter the stroke survivor's condition, keep them moving and active. One day, Mommy was taking her time riding the stationary bike when her sense of humor popped in. She started to pedal faster and faster, because she was excited that she was still coordinated and was doing something that others could do.

With great zeal Mommy shouted, "WHHHEEEEE! I'll meet you down at the corner, girlfriend!"

Wow, she was really riding that bike. Her headsets were on; the music was blaring, and she was laughing. I joined in on the fun.

"Mommy, slow down. Now make a right turn. Now make a left."

I laughed as Mommy acted out every point of direction I gave her. It was great fun.

"Wow! You went for seventeen minutes today. That's great. Now it's my turn."

I rode with a funny hat on for twenty minutes. I rolled off the bike exhausted, and Mommy laughed at me. I had to stay in shape too. Panting, I made my way to the chair to sit down.

Daddy came into the room. "What are you guys doing? You're having too much fun in here."

"You go ahead, Cliff," Mommy said. "Take your ride for the day, brah" (short for brother).

Daddy got on the bike and, like me, ended up out of breath, but he rode longer than the both of us. That made Mommy feel good about herself. She was the only one not out of breath.

Riding the Rainbow

We loved when Daddy joined in. My dad is the greatest. After the epic bike workout, Daddy kissed Mommy and headed out of the room. She and I hugged and drank from the cold water bottles Daddy got for us.

Mommy looked at me. "Thank you."

Still a little winded but grateful, I replied, "No, Mommy. Thank you! You get an E for effort! High five!" (Smack)

CHAPTER 22

Things to Remember

In most cases, people achieve what they can achieve, what they *believe* they can achieve, and what *you* believe they can achieve. Sometimes you must be the one who has confidence in their ability when they don't have it themselves. Keep in mind, things can be easy or hard. No matter what, celebrate everything! E for effort, right? Excellent! Here are some things to remember that will help you with this process.

When problems come up, don't always ignore them.

Many times, you have to meet the challenges head on, directly, but do it with a pillow, not a stone. Whenever possible, remind the stroke survivor that they're like other people in many ways. Some of the things they do and feel silly about are the same things we all do and feel silly about.

Even though the survivor may look normal, talk normal and even walk normal, remember that they had a stroke. This is very important.

The effects from the stroke may cause them to say and do things that are, shall we say, out of character. Be gentle, compassionate and understanding and try not to take it personally. My sister was an expert with this.

My sister insisted Mommy walk by herself because my sister *believed* she could. And guess what? My mother could do it. It was only when I came around and felt sorry for her or overprotective that Mommy reached out for me with a sad face. "Help me, Janice."

Most of the time, I couldn't resist. I helped her every time unless Sharon was around. When my sister was around, she'd get on me if I helped Mommy.

"No, Janice. Don't you move. She can do it herself." Sharon encouraged her with tough love. "Mommy, you can do this!"

And Mommy would do it. She could walk. It was like seeing a miracle happen right before our eyes every time.

Daddy was a sucker too. If my mother looked at him with sad helpless eyes, he couldn't help himself. He helped her without hesitation. It was Sharon and the therapists who showed my mother that she could do the impossible and be independent. It was hard for me, Daddy and my brothers to be tough. But, again, everyone had value, meaning and a role to play.

Mommy loved seeing Clifton. When he came by, Mommy shook with excitement. She always said she loved all her children equally, but there was something special about her firstborn. This was processed with no jealousy or envy from any of us. Mommy and Daddy always had enough love for all.

Mommy admired and saw herself in Sharon. Sharon's beautiful and talented and is a wonderful artist, singer and fantastic mother like Mommy. She's strong like Mommy too. Sharon's training and education as a registered nurse was invaluable to Mommy's healing journey. She was always in good hands.

Ronald, Donald and their wives were instrumental with their medical backgrounds. This was priceless when it came to helping with Mommy. Like Michael and Clifton, when the boys came by the house, and Mommy cooed over them. "Oooohhh, I love my babies. My boys! They are so handsome! I'm going to marry each one of them!"

Michael was our gentle giant, six-foot-five and Mommy's baby boy. Michael helped however he could, even if it was just standing there looking good and laughing.

All the spouses of my siblings played important and special roles. From medical advice, to fixing things around the house, to bringing the grandchildren over, or just being there so that we could play spades, eat blue crabs, and have fun. They were all—and still are—very special and precious.

Whether you are the survivor, the caregiver, friend or spouse, don't count yourself out. Don't let others cancel you out and make sure you don't cancel anyone out either. The more the merrier, as long as everyone remains positive. Embrace life with courage, pride and humor whenever possible.

Finally, if you can, give each other a lot of affection and hands-on loving. I love to hug people, and I loved to toss Mommy around the bed when I was putting her to sleep like she was on a rollercoaster.

"I love that, Janice!" She laughed as I gently bounced her body up and down while getting her on her side position to sleep.

It's imperative to eliminate as much stress as you can for the stroke survivor and for yourself. Make rest a priority. When my mother didn't get enough rest, she was prone to having seizures because of the scarring on the brain caused by the stroke. It looked a lot like an epileptic episode.

When this happened, we simply held her and reassured her that the convulsions were almost over. Mommy was put on Dilantin, an anti-convulsant. This medication can be tricky. Too much in their system may bring on the side effects like skin rashes or sleeping too much. Too little in their system, the seizures could come back more frequently and stronger.

Mommy was fully aware of her surroundings when she was having a seizure. She fearfully looked into our eyes to find comfort. Survivors will also use your body language and facial expressions as indicators of how bad the situation might be or how bad it might look. Remain calm, comforting and soothing. Smile if you can.

Comforting phrases go a long way to soothe a person in crisis.

"It's okay. Oh yeah, we've been here before. Relax. It'll go away. Yeah, I got ya. I'm right here. It's almost over." Our father rubbed her back during a troublesome episode.

We copied behaviors we saw Dad model beautifully. We learned how to comfort Mommy and her nerves.

Here's a snapshot of how we debriefed after one of her seizures:

Janice: "How did you feel about that seizure, Mommy? Was it as strong as the last one?"

Mommy: "No. it wasn't as strong as the last one. I think I did pretty good with this one."

Janice: "Yeah, I agree. You did really well."

Daddy: "Yep. I think it's one of those things we're going to have to learn to live with for the time being, baby. Remember the doctor said it's not harming you, so that's good."

Mommy: "Right, Cliff."

Daddy: "You did great, baby. You were calm and kept control of your breathing."

Mommy: "Yep, it's just one of those things that I'll have to handle."

These debriefing sessions were another example of respecting a stroke survivor and allowing them to build their own sense of agency and empowerment. (Side note: I also noticed Mommy's seizures coincided with the full moon. Just an observation).

After a seizure, no matter who was with her, we'd kiss Mommy and hug her. We always made it a habit to look her straight in her eyes and say, "You did great, Mommy. You're fine. Now, let's get some rest, okay?"

"Sounds good." Mommy smiled and thanked God for helping us make it through another hurdle.

Riding the Rainbow

The gentle massage will help them to physically calm down, feel protected and safe. Make sure the survivor doesn't hit themselves with anything and doesn't fall on anything. Additionally, make sure they don't bite their tongues in the midst of the seizure. After the seizure, the person may be tired for a couple of days. Let them sleep. Then when the time is right, acknowledge and talk about what happened.

We found Valerian tea or capsules helped Mommy to sleep and stay calm, organic aloe vera juice and chlorophyll helped her stay healthy, and a little Irish Bristol Cream never hurt her from time to time. We used an herbalist in partnership with our regular doctor. All beneficial.

CHAPTER 23

Don't Miss It

Small miracles can happen right before your eyes. Each day may contain a blessing or a miracle. Make sure you don't miss it!

After a few years of little to no movement of Mommy's left leg, foot and toes, a miracle happened.

I was giving Mommy her shower. "Mommy, can you relax while I wash your back? You're tightening up."

She laughed and her stomach that had six children (twins at that) jiggled like Jello. Great muscle control! I look at her belly, poked it, and like the Pillsbury Dough Boy, it jiggled again.

She giggled.

"What's that, Mommy?"

"Look, Janice!" Mommy made her stomach jump up and down using her muscles. The jiggling was even more pronounced when she laughed.

"Keep still, Mommy. We're in the shower. We have to be careful."

We continued to laugh.

"Mommy, be careful. I don't want you to fall!"

Suddenly her left toes tightened up! Our eyes poked out!

I watched Mommy's left leg, foot and toes curl up as she's laughed. It could have been parts of her body connecting with her brain. In the moment, I thought about what I was seeing. *Is this a miracle?* I saw something the doctors said would never happen. It had been over three years since the stroke.

"Mommy, your toes are curling up!"

"I know! Oh shhhh . . . Janice."

"Can you do it again?" I wondered if her brain could intentionally tell her toes to curl up. She did it again!

"Look, Janice! Look!"

"I know! Oh ssshhhh . . . Let's get out of this shower!"

We yelled, laughed, clapped, and thanked the good Lord for the miracle. At that moment, at that very second, with the curling of her toes, Mommy was a brand-new woman with new hopes! It felt like a miracle. It was a miracle.

From that day on, we continued to work the left side every single day and every single day, her left side came back a little more. Mommy never stopped smiling, and the improvements just kept coming. I smile now, just thinking about it.

Riding the Rainbow

Speaking of the bathroom. As a caregiver, you may have to help your loved one with toileting tasks. If they can do it themselves, let them. Then take a moment to check to make sure everything is clean. Even amid basic tasks like bathing and toileting, there can be many challenging and stressful situations. There can also be the occasional blessings and miracles. Embrace and savor them all. Our blessings and miracles included Mommy's left side coming back wonderfully. That allowed her to do more with both arms, legs and hands. Isn't God good?

CHAPTER 24

And Don't Forget

Therapy is important for recovery, and it must begin quickly after the stroke is diagnosed. Therapy—intense therapy—can determine the success of a stroke survivor's recovery. Occupational, speech and physical therapy are very beneficial to improvement. The effectiveness of these processes can sometimes predict how well and how fast an individual will recover and heal. If allowable and doable, I also recommend emotional and mental health therapy so that the survivor can talk to someone outside of the family if needed. Whatever affordable help the family can attain is invaluable. I say try it.

Be sure the stroke survivor is comfortable with their therapist—physically, emotionally, spiritually and psychologically. Be sure the caregiver and anyone else who is helping the survivor is also comfortable with the therapist *and* the facilities. If there isn't a level of being comfortable on any aspect, talk to your doctor about other available options. Don't always assume things will get better, or the survivor will get used to it. Talk about it, address it and change it if needed, without hesitation.

Remember, because it is hard work and the therapist pushes the survivor to do things, doesn't mean the work they are doing is bad for them. At the same time, you don't want the survivor to stop before they get started because of conflicts and uncomfortable challenges. Address the conflicts and challenges head on, then decide what is best for your loved one and their recovery. Be sure to make decisions *with* the stroke survivor involved.

Mommy worked well with therapists who were physically strong, taller than her, compassionate, soft spoken, encouraging, believed in a loving God and displayed an obvious element of optimism with a sense of humor. Like Daddy! A therapist may not have all these characteristics, which goes back to the importance of everyone being a part of the support system.

At one time or another, my father, sister and I became Mommy's fulltime physical therapist in partnership with the professionals. This worked out well, because we were able to continue the therapy outside of the facilities. Now, catch this nugget; it's important.

The therapists cannot do it alone.

The most effective therapy, in our opinion, is one that involves family members in the physical therapy sessions which are continued at home. We knew Mommy's ways, so we were able to navigate through some challenges with a keen insight to her personality. Physical therapy can get you started, but it's up to the survivor *and* the family to keep the true momentum going.

Physical therapy can be done right where the survivor is sitting, standing or laying down. Every chance we got, we exercised Mommy's body. We did leg exercises, arm exercises and simple movements of the body while she was still in bed, hoping to reconnect to her muscle memory. Whatever the stroke survivors state of mobility is, keep them moving, keep the body and the mind active.

If the survivor doesn't want to get better, it may be difficult for you or the therapist to provide aid. Sometimes, they become depressed. This can be paralyzing. Everything will cease when this happens. They won't eat, laugh, go to therapy—nothing. They will simply exist, which deters the healing and recovery processes. You must do your best to get to know each other, hopefully before the stroke, and grow together after the stroke.

Please, please communicate with your doctor and the medical team; it's key to the plan for holistic wellness for your loved one. My mother had a very positive attitude, sense of humor and a strong mental and emotional foundation built upon her faith in God. Consequently, and fortunately, she brought all of this with her when she faced the stroke. This gave us a great foundation to start the healing process with our mother. For your family, it could be another form of spirituality, meditation, music, sports, food . . . whatever keeps the peace and sanity in your life, keep it going.

If you don't have something positive to work with from the beginning, start working on that right now. If you can't do it, find someone who can, until you learn how to take the first step toward a positive recovery. A positive recovery to me is a recovery that brings the family closer and keeps the stroke survivor alive and kicking spiritually and physically. The rest will, hopefully, follow.

Of course, you can always read this book as many times as you'd like for inspiration and actionable tips. Hopefully, doing this will bring a smile to your face and give you the energy needed to go forward optimistically.

I must also share that things were not always done with a smile and positivity during Mommy's healing journey. One time when I was still living in Atlanta, Daddy called me to talk to Mommy. This was when Mommy first had her stroke. She was sad and a little depressed that day.

"Hey, Mommy! How are you doing? I hear you're not feeling very well. What's wrong?" I asked her.

"When is this all going to be over? When will I be normal again," she asked as she cried over the phone.

Feeling her heart and speaking from my faith, I said, "I understand, Mommy. Don't you worry. Things will get better. I promise, okay? Just hang in there, okay? Things will get better. I'll be there to see you soon, okay?"

"Yes," she quietly responded.

"Tell me what else is going on before I start singing to you."

"Oh Lawd, Janice. Please don't."

We both laughed and continued to laugh as we made light conversation. I did not hang up until Mommy felt and sounded better. I was so grateful that Daddy called me to help. It's through trials and tribulations that you discover the blessing and purpose God has on your life to help others.

As far as I know and as far as Daddy can remember, Mommy never complained or cried again, although one never knows what happened in the quiet of night when everyone was sleeping. We spent the rest of our time over the years working on getting better. All we can do is try to be there when sadness or depression shows up. All things are possible through Christ who strengthens us.

I'm sure you've heard that a spoonful of sugar can help medicine go down, right? Well, that's not always the case. The administration of medication can be problematic, especially if you are taking medicinal pills and herbal supplements. The number of pills and how many times you have to swallow can add up. Depending on the count, getting all of them down can be taxing. Let your loved one take their time and move through it cautiously. Mommy got tired of taking so many pills. She didn't take many prescription pills, but she took quite a few vitamins and supplements to support her overall health.

Daddy came up with the idea of Mommy drinking chlorophyll and organic aloe vera juice after doing some research. These are great for the body. We believed that by combining natural and medicinal remedies was the reason Mommy was only on insulin for a short period of time after her stroke, along with exercise of course, a positive attitude and a healthy diet. We hired a naturopathic doctor who was also a traditional doctor to help with this process.

A healthy diet doesn't have to be tasteless. I learned to cook from Mommy, and we believed in seasoning things right. I didn't stop this practice when I began to fix three meals a day for the four plus years I was helping my parents as her caregiver. She ate well and stayed healthy. Mommy didn't pass away from the things she ate. She passed away from an infection she contracted while her kidneys were being tested in the hospital. This was something no one could have predicted.

So, encourage your loved one to eat well and not to be shy with the seasonings like garlic, ginger and pepper. Everyone needs to watch salt, sugar and processed foods.

And then there is the "doctor." I put doctor in quotations because our doctor was more than a doctor. He was like a part of the family, a friend who seemed to care for my mother as much as we did. He was compassionate, intelligent and proactive. On top of everything, the good doctor communicated well and thoroughly.

Dr. O.T. Adcock took the time to get to know my mother as a person. He was generous with the preventive measures he suggested. With beautiful bedside manners, a great sense of humor, an abundance of kindness, thoughtfulness and caring, our visits to him were always reassuring, and that says a great deal.

Our family truly believed that Dr. Adcock, who worked at Riverside Medical Center in Hampton, Virginia, off Mercury Boulevard, was heaven sent. We couldn't have asked for a better caregiver in this capacity. We believed he was and is the best. Dr. Adcock, thank you for everything. We love you so very much. You will always be in our thoughts and in our prayers forever and ever. Amen.

Daddy and I recorded every single visit. In fact, we not only recorded the appointments, but Daddy also wrote notes on each visit. This was important because, no matter who came around or what doctor or herbalist we spoke to, we always had a running and thorough medical record about Mommy. We even kept up with when she had seizures. Daddy posted a list of all the medications, herbs and supplements Mommy was taking on the refrigerator so, at a glance, everyone was informed.

Riding the Rainbow

Our family prays that your family will find a doctor that you feel comfortable working with as we did. It's a wonderful gift during the recovery process to have a doctor who cares for the stroke survivor and continues to be positive, yet realistic. Remember, if you're not comfortable with your doctor, look for other options.

CHAPTER 25

Dignity

The women in Mommy's family prided themselves on being ladylike with beautiful arches in their feet and shapely figures, great lovers to their husbands, great chefs in the kitchen, and extremely intelligent and funny. They were outspoken and believed women could do whatever they set their minds to, whether they decided to be fulltime mothers, career women outside of the home, or both. No matter their choice, they always had wonderful men to support them and who helped take care of the household and whatever they needed or desired. They were dignified.

One of the most challenging things about recovering from a stroke is keeping one's dignity, pride, self-esteem and self-worth intact. A sense of dignity supports the self-respect of the survivor. It's important to recognize their capacities and ambitions and take care not to do anything that undermines their healing and positive mindset. This includes, but is not limited to, respect for what they can do, who they are, and the life they've lived. It's seen as a central part of quality in care work.

Mommy always liked to look her best. She had a routine before the stroke, and Daddy made sure that the same routine was uninterrupted as much as possible after the stroke. Every Thursday, Mommy got her hair done by Miss Gwen and her nails done by Miss Kim. Whenever possible, I laid Mommy down in a bathtub and let her wash herself and relax. She loved feeling, smelling and looking clean.

She had shoes to walk in and shoes to look good in while lounging in the house. She wore tennis shoes when she was walking, but if she was sitting in church or at an event, we switched out the tennis shoes for dress shoes once she was seated. Even though it was a considerate gesture when friends of the family offered to take Mommy to the bathroom, we made sure someone in her immediate family took her whenever possible. Think about it. Although it may be more convenient, no one wants everyone in the world to see their hiney in the bathroom. What would you consider appropriate for yourself? Give that same consideration to your loved one.

Another way to maintain pride and dignity is allowing the stroke survivor to be productive in their home and in the community. Mommy and I started writing this book to help the community, for example.

She had a beautiful complexion; she never used harsh soap on her face, drank lots of water and got out in the sun whenever she could for natural vitamin D. She maintained this ritual before and after the stroke. She assisted on bathing herself, setting the meal menus, brushing her teeth, washing her face and cleaning the bathroom sink until she told me she was ready. At that time, I walked her back to her room where she put on lotion, deodorant, perfume, and of course, lipstick. She also combed her hair in front of a mobile vanity mirror that sat on a tray table. She helped me prepare food for meals, folded clothes and decided what she was going to wear. She loved bright colors, so she dressed sunny and bright.

Mommy also continued to give her input on what Daddy should wear. For my entire life, I saw Daddy get his clothes together, which usually consisted of a shirt, tie, pants, belt, shoes, socks and sometimes a hat. He picked things out and turned to Mommy. "Hey, baby, what do you think about this tie with this shirt?"

She gave her opinion, and Daddy made the changes if required. He always wanted to look good, especially for her.

I don't remember Mommy ever wearing something that was inappropriate. They dressed for each other, and without knowing it, they also dressed for their children. Role models of self-respect. I always loved that about my mother and father. As amazing as they were individually, they always humbled themselves to the love and grace of each other.

Side note: this is totally subjective. There are varied levels of self-respect that parents teach their children. We pass no judgment. What counts is the heart.

On the other hand, it was a good thing Mommy picked out her own clothes, because mistakes could be made by her caregivers when we were in a hurry. I can't tell you the number of times we had her shoes on the wrong foot or had forgotten to put her underwear on. On one occasion, I kept seeing Mommy's cash fall to the floor. I picked it up, and being old school, she put it back in her brassiere. Still, time after time, it kept falling to the ground until I asked, "Mommy, why in the world can you not hold onto that money?"

"Because you forgot to put my bra on!"

Now, that was funny! Once we put her in high water pants that came to her ankles. Poor Mommy. Surprisingly, she never got mad at our mistakes. It made for great opportunities to have a good laugh or two. It's so therapeutic to laugh, right?

Mommy picked out and put on her own jewelry whenever possible. Daddy always helped with her earrings. She vacuumed while standing or sitting, dusted the table she always sat next to in the living room and cleared and wiped off the dining room table for dinner.

To keep her dignity when it came to taking pills out in public and at home, I bought her two very nice, ivory pill boxes from the 1920s or so. This way, every time she went to take her pills, the classiness of it stayed, rather than the reminder that something may not be right.

To keep the stroke survivor's general disposition and healthy glow, please don't keep them cloistered in the house or a room. Even if they do nothing but sit, get them out into the sunshine if it's okay with the doctor. Sitting on a porch or at the beach were two of Mommy's favorite settings.

Keeping a collection of books, puzzles, magazines or newspapers available is ideal to keep the survivor's mind engaged and attitude buoyant. This will enlighten the conversations as much as a nice cup of tea or glass of lemonade. Even a little wine here and there will keep the mind stimulated and sharp (red is probably a good choice). These small things will also keep the stroke survivor involved in a normal society and way of life. We all need that from time to time, don't we?

In addition to Miss Kim doing Mommy's nails and Miss Gwen doing her hair, a small circle of women surrounded my mother. Mrs. Shirley Tyler, Mrs. Richardson, Miss Chastain, and of course, Miss Rosetta and so many others were just wonderful. We thank you.

Before Sharon moved to Alabama, she cared for Mommy along with Miss Jackson, Miss Rosetta, Miss Joyce and Mrs. Trudi. With each day and challenge, Sharon never gave up on Mommy. Mommy fell a few times, which made her nervous. But Sharon knew what Mommy could do and, through the pushbacks, the pouts and the stubbornness, used tough love that she learned from our mother. Mommy regained her mobility. Up and down the hall, in and out of the bathroom, to and from her bed, repeatedly Sharon and Mommy exercised self-empowerment. A can-do attitude and boot camp—Sharon style!

Once Mommy got to that point, all I had to do was let her hold one of my fingers or my hand to boost her confidence, and she walked without a problem.

I will always remember a special moment when Mommy looked at Sharon, pulled her close and said she was sorry for all the times she was impatient and that she loved her. She repeatedly said, "Thank you," while hugging and kissing her.

Being the beautiful person my sister is and has always been, Sharon knew Mommy felt those things, but I'm sure it was nice to hear it during those challenging times. Thank you, Mommy.

Finally, in addition to my immediate and extended family members, I want to tell you about another set of angels who came into our lives during this healing journey. I want to thank all the wonderful people at my mother's job at Fort Monroe, Virginia, where she worked in civil service. Invited by my father, they donated enough sick time to Mommy that she didn't lose pay for two years and retired with full benefits.

A diverse cadre of people gave their time, prayers and love to my mother. If it were not for her colleagues, the beginning of this journey would have been rough indeed. We love you all, and we will never forget what a group of splendid people did for one person, our mother, out of love. Pure and simple, out of love and compassion, you gave from your heart and now our family has, continuously, tried to pass that same love onto others over the years. Thank you for your soulful and loving example.

Riding the Rainbow

Dignity is one of those things that is felt, worn and seen. It marries itself to the direct identity of who a person is to themselves and to the world. Just like hope, it's a key component to the very existence of a human being as a member of society who refuses to be kept in the shadows after a stroke. And like hope, when this dignity is felt, when this dignity is taken care of just like their physical bodies, their emotions and the clothes they wear, it is one of the most valuable and most important components of a person's introduction and reintroduction to the world. While they may have lost a lot, there is no reason they should ever lose their dignity. If it, by chance, is lost, I implore and encourage you to step up to this honorable position of helping them to find it again and be the safekeeper of it all.

Chapter 26

My Daddy, Mommy's Baby: Lessons from My Father

I wanted to make this last chapter about my daddy, or Mommy's "baby," as she called him. My parents were married for almost forty-two years before my mother passed in 2002. Other than God and Jesus Christ, my father is the best man I know. After him, my brothers.

Daddy is such a good father, husband, friend, man, Christian and American. I had to give him his own chapter, even though it would be easy for me to write an entire book on him and the goodness of his heart. I hope, through the reading of this book, you have gained an idea of how much of a blessing he has been to us.

The men surrounding Mommy throughout her life were funny, intelligent and hardworking. They always had good jobs (sometimes more than one), were well educated and took care of the women in their lives as providers. While they worked jobs and built careers, some extended their education attaining a master's or a doctorate degree.

All the men, including my father, were what some people call a man's man. They knew how to fix any and everything in the house, on cars or lawn mowers and were just all-around handy. You name it, they could fix it. And if they didn't know how, they gathered around in a circle with a libation or two and talked about the problem until they came up with a solution. They believed in taking care of their wives, and the women were happy to take care of their men.

Daddy always took care of Mommy and our family but also Mommy's family and his mother and father when he became a man. He served his country in the Army for twenty-one years, retiring as a lieutenant colonel. Then he retired after nineteen years in federal civil service, all while teaching college math courses and taking care of our mother. He was an athlete from high school through college—football, wrestling and baseball. A great student, Daddy skipped grades to begin college at a very young age . . . I think around fifteen. Daddy is handsome, kind, funny and strong. He is everything! He is the type of father who fixed our bikes and everyone else's bike in the neighborhood.

He believed in discipline, hard work, a positive attitude and kindness for everyone you meet, so none of us really met any strangers. He and Mommy held Bible study in thirteen different living rooms before I turned fourteen, because being a military brat, that's about the number of times we had to move in the first fourteen years of my life.

We always said our grace, the Pledge of Allegiance to the Flag and our prayers. We apologized and loved our sister, brothers and others. Mommy and Daddy were always family-oriented, so it was easy for me to decide to move home and take care of family. I thank my parents for these wonderful traits, ones that they passed onto their children.

My daddy also held the admiration and respect of both men and women. Being from the country where you had to fix things on your own, whenever I had car problems, he'd tell me to put the phone up to the engine of my car, so he could hear it and tell me what might be going on, like Goober or Gomer on the *Andy Griffith Show,* one of his favorites. He's also a woman's man because of the way he loved and treated my mother and his family; women and men alike admired their relationship. From the day we were born, our family always came first.

Mommy was Daddy's love, and the children were the offspring of this love affair. But Mommy and Daddy were more than husband and wife. They were buddies, pals and best friends. I say this because when Mommy first had her stroke, Daddy was there every night, every morning and every afternoon, keeping her comfortable and safe. When it was time for therapy, Daddy stayed with her in the hospital room in a chair or on a cot and went with her to every therapy session until I took over, and he went back to work fulltime.

When Mommy was released from the hospital and went home, Daddy, this big man, every man's man, showered and bathed her, dried her off, applied lotion to her body, helped get her clothes out and dressed her. This meant that he had to get up at five or five-thirty in the morning to do all of this before he went to work Monday through Friday. He called throughout the day to tell her he loved her and to check on her.

Daddy hugged and kissed Mommy all the time while telling her she looked so pretty. Then at night, this big, masculine, six-feet two-inches, two hundred and thirty pounds of a man rolled Mommy's hair, dressed her in nightclothes and tucked her into bed. Now, that's after he got her some Irish Bristol Cream (one of her favorites) or sugar-free cookies.

Throughout the night, when Mommy got up to use the bathroom, Daddy was at his post next to the bed; he was there to tuck her back into bed. This meant Daddy wasn't really getting any rest. His sleep was always interrupted, but he never complained. He didn't want Mommy to ever feel like he wasn't there for her.

When Daddy had business trips, if he could, he took Mommy. Every single weekend was spent making her happy, doing what she wanted to do. Daddy said he did it because he loved her and was doing what he was supposed to do. My parents always said one of the keys to a good marriage is to love the Lord, love your family and out love your spouse each and every day.

Every morning, my parents would wake up and think of how they could out love each other. What a wonderful way of not just saying you love someone but performing that love with a grateful heart! This was a constant in our family—serving and loving with a grateful heart.

When it was time for us to move, Mommy had the house and the kids packed up. "Okay, where are we going next, Cliff-baby?"

She made our constant moving an adventure and fun, so we never complained. They were a great match—equally yoked.

Daddy never used Mommy's illness as an excuse to "act crazy," as Mommy called it. She meant hanging out at the clubs, flirting with other women, stop coming home, not participating in the daily activities of the home and family, etc. My dad was there every time we needed him.

Once Daddy married Mommy, the only wild days he saw were experienced with her sitting on his lap, watching over each other at every party. They had an enduring passion that they kept alive their entire life together and a passion my father kept alive even after Mommy's stroke. She was always riding shotgun with her favorite guy!

Mommy also continued to dote on my dad. When it was time for him to come home, Mommy heard the roar of the twin pipes of his red Dakota truck and, literally and physically, pushed me out of the way so she could get to the living room to greet him. Her body shook with excitement when she said, "There he is! Daddy's home, Janice! Move! My baby's here! My baby's here! Come on, baby! Oh! You smell so good! I can smell you from here! Move, Janice!"

I laughed at her excitement.

When he came through the door, Mommy got louder! "There he is! There he is! Hhhmmmm, baby, come here! You look sooooo good and smell so good! Come here so I can give you a kiss!"

Daddy smiled, laughed and headed up the stairs to get all that loving Mommy had waiting for him. He smiled while Mommy kissed him all over his face, hugging him around the neck. Now *that* is passion! And it's probably why they had six kids when they originally didn't want any! It's all good, because it's all God!

The reason I tell you this part of their story is because it's really important to remember that when one spouse has a stroke, it absolutely affects the other spouse. So, keep the romance and love going anyway you can and for as long as you can. You're in it together.

My daddy is truly heaven sent. Through the ups and downs, my parents stayed true to each other, loved each other and stayed committed to each other. I'm sure there were challenges, but they chose to stick with it, to ride it out together. That's the most important lesson here. Stay together so you both can make it through . . . together. When you have doubts, do like my dad always said to do: always make a decision you can live with.

Their type of loving served as the type of relationship we wanted to emulate, as their children. I think it is good to remember that when a spouse or partner has had a stroke, your children are still watching and learning from your behavior. If you choose, it is an opportunity to show your children how healthy and loving partnerships really work. No matter the scenario, remember, you are still role models - teaching your children what to do and what not to do. Unfortunately, as life would have it, some partnerships make it through while others don't. It is not easy, either way.

In my parents case, when people would try to give Daddy compliments about how well he was taking care of Mommy, he simply said, "I'm doing what I'm supposed to do. I love my baby." How precious is that? Amazing.

I want to make a quick note of another special moment involving my father. During my mother's recovery, my father attacked prostate cancer that was trying to attack him. I saw Mommy be there for him, taking care of him by making sure he took his medicine on time, ate on time and drank lots of water.

I'll never forget when I made a pallet for myself on the floor next to their bed while Daddy was recovering. Throughout the night, Daddy needed special attention with his dressing, medication, repositioning and other things to help with his recovery. Mommy also needed me to watch over her since Daddy couldn't at the time, so I decided to go old school and just camp out on the floor. That way they didn't have to yell for me.

I don't think I slept for an entire week, but I didn't feel tired. I wanted to stay on top of my game and take care of my parents, and I loved every minute of it. Caring for them was such a blessing for me. To this day, one of my fondest memories is loving on my mother and father and feeling honored to be there for them, like they had been there for their children our entire lives. I was right there, at their feet, ready to be called. Amen.

By the way, Daddy beat the cancer.

Now back to my father. Daddy always saw himself as somewhat of a dream weaver in Mommy's life. He thought it was his duty since day one to love and cherish Mommy and make her dreams come true. Since the stroke, one of my mother's dreams was to have a ranch-style home. A single-level house so she wouldn't have to deal with anymore stairs. Well, guess what? Daddy moved Mommy into a new ranch, designed as handicap accessible.

The way I remember the story is that the original owner of the house had suffered a stroke and had the house built for handicap accessibility in all ways. Within two months of moving in, the owner improved and was able to move out and WHAM! The house was put up for sale. Mommy and Daddy bought it, moved in and began an even more interactive way of living, despite the stroke. It was an answer to their prayers and the manifestation of Mommy's dreams! How good is God, I ask you? Amazing!

The showers, cabinets, doors, hallways, doorways, sinks, bars, rails—everything was designed to help someone get around who was physically challenged or used a wheelchair. I had never seen my mother so happy than when she moved into that house!

At first, when she was wheelin' and dealin' in her motorized wheelchair, she went so fast, she scraped walls and knocked over chairs. We only said, "Slow your roll!"

Mommy was happy and independent. She was back to being herself. She laughed and went faster!

This was the first time in seven years Mommy was able to go anywhere in her house without assistance. After her morning routine, she went to her sunroom, opened the blinds and sat at the breakfast table awaiting the meal Daddy was fixing. Or Mommy got a cold drink from the refrigerator, put the dirty cup in the dishwasher, throw trash away, dust off the furniture or look through the cupboards for a snack. Sometimes she was wheelin' and dealin' just because she could.

She could now do all the things she did before the stroke but couldn't after because we lived in a split-level house with narrow hallways and openings and high cabinets and so forth. Once in the new home, Mommy had greater independence and felt empowered and powerful. She was Mommy times ten, Vi, Viola Collins and Baby again. And boy, was she sailing! Riding the rainbow on cloud nine, ten, and eleven! Flying higher than she had flown in the last seven years. Smiling wider, broader and brighter.

The new home allowed Mommy to find a new wind beneath her wings. A bold breeze carried her to many pots of gold and helped her glide through the days. Up, up and away to a colorful, beautiful, bright, rainbow journey. What a wonderful gift. What a wonderful woman. What a wonderful husband. What a wonderful father and man.

Thank you, Daddy, for that beautiful dream of a home and more.

Riding the Rainbow

When I look back on how Mommy was taken care of, I realize she was cared for like she had always been cared for—like a queen. We loved on her each and every day. The way I see it, we returned to Mommy all the love she had given each of us throughout our lives. All the protection, caring and nurturing gifts she shared with all seven of us, she got back seven-fold! What a blessing for *us* to have given all of it back to her! She had earned it and deserved every ounce.

Now, I want to turn my attention just to you, the reader. I want to thank you for taking the time to read our book. Whether you were reading it for yourself or to a survivor of a stroke, whether you are a caregiver or simply reading it for curiosity or pleasure, I hope you have smiled a little more.

While you may not know if a pot of gold awaits you at end of your rainbow, there may be pots of gold awaiting you *on* your journey. There is the journey, and there is how you face your journey and your mindset during the adventure. Make it positive and don't let the grass grow underneath your feet.

Also remember to go easy on yourself. You can only do your best. Remember that no one is perfect, and it's not always going to be easy, but you are uniquely built for the journey. And while misery loves company, you don't have to accept the invitation. So, buckle in for safety and enjoy the ride. If you ever feel down, try one of my mother's tricks and keep looking up!

Dear Readers,

We wish you victories, love, support, better health, courage and beautiful moments as you ride through the storm(s). We pray you find your own special wind that takes you gently on a rainbow ride full of bright and beautiful colors. Keep moving!

God bless you! We're pulling for you and always praying for you.

Off you go!

Love,

The Collins family

Lessons From Our Father Who Art In Heaven

The Spirituality of It ALL

I want to tell you a few short stories about my experiences in how the Father works on Earth as it is in Heaven. First, a sequence of events that led to a blessing.

First Sequence: Mommy's phone call

One Friday when I got home from seeing my parents, about two weeks before Mommy's passing, Mommy called to say thank you.

"Hey, Mommy! What's going on?"

"Nothing. I just want to say thank you, Janice."

"Okay . . . for what?"

"For everything! Thank you so much! Do you hear me?"

"Yes, Mommy! I hear you. You're welcome, shortay. But what's going on? I just saw you and you're acting a little weird, weirdo," I said as I laughed.

"I just want to say thank you. Thank you. Thank you! I love you, Janice! Hear me? I love you! Thank you! For everything!"

"Okay, Mommy, you're welcome. Are you okay? Do you want me to come back over?"

"Thank you, baby."

"Okay. You're welcome, Mommy. I'll call you later to check on you, Okay? I love you."

"I love you too"

After hearing our conversation, my housemate came into the kitchen. "Is everything okay with your mom?"

"Yeah. I think she's okay. She just wanted to say thank you to me, I guess. I'm going to call and check back on her later."

I thought the conversation was a little strange but just figured Mommy was having a moment. That's all. When I called back later in the evening to check on her and ask her about the weird phone call, she said she didn't know what I was talking about. She said she didn't make any such call.

The next week, Mommy went to the hospital to get her kidneys checked.

Second Sequence: Was it a Dream?

Daddy was in the home office while Mommy was taking a nap in the bedroom in their new home. Being so tired from working and taking care of Mommy, Daddy fell asleep at the computer. After a few minutes, he jumped up, thinking he heard Mommy calling his name, saying she needed him. Daddy ran so fast through the house that his shoulder went through a wall when he stumbled a bit. He brushed it off and ran to the bedroom.

"Yes, baby? What is it?" Daddy asked.

Mommy looked puzzled. "What are you talking about, Cliff?"

"You told me to come help you. You were calling my name."

"No, I wasn't, silly."

"Are you sure you're okay, baby?"

"Yes, Cliff. I am. Thank you," Mommy said.

Third Sequence: 3:45-4:15 and The Cloud

Before Mommy went in for her kidney procedure, a few other things happened that may have been a little unsettling when they happened but brought comfort to me in my time of need.

When my parents moved to their new home in Yorktown, they still owned the home in Hampton that we had lived in since I was around thirteen. It was my childhood home where we lived the longest as a family. Our home in Hampton was about two miles from a townhouse I was renting with a childhood friend. Anytime I wanted to feel close to my mother, instead of driving twenty to twenty-five minutes to the new house, I got on my motorcycle and headed to the beach. Laying on the sand, looking up at the stars, I felt close to God, which meant I also felt close to my mother.

This changed when, for the next month or so—I don't remember the time duration exactly—I would awaken at three forty-five in the morning, get into my mother's Honda Accord that I drove for work, and drive to our old house. I would get out of the car, look around the house, the front and backyard, then get back into my car and return to the townhouse. I did this over and over and over. Three forty-five every morning, I had a spiritual feeling, almost a push, to go to our old house. Once in a while, the time would adjust to four fifteen in the morning, but I would do the exact same thing. I told Mommy about it.

"It's been so weird. I always wake up at three forty-five or four fifteen in the morning. I don't know what it means. Do you?" I asked her one day.

"No. I don't know, girlfriend. Maybe they're the winning lottery ticket numbers!"

"Maybe! I'm going to play those numbers. I'll break you off a piece if I win." We had a good laugh over it.

Besides the time element, the other thing I remembered was the intense feeling that something was just not right. I began to pray. I continued to visit our old home in the middle of the night. As I got closer to the house, I felt a sense of uneasiness, like someone was trying to break into the house or something. Since we still owned the house, I thought perhaps someone was trying to steal something that was left inside, but I never went in.

During one of my visits, when I started to look for clues or signs as to why I felt this strange feeling, I noticed an ominous cloud over our house that I hadn't noticed before. It was blue, gray, a little dark and centered directly above our house like in the movie *Close Encounters of the Third Kind*. I didn't hear or see a spaceship, so I knew that wasn't it. So, again, I got back into my car and returned to my townhouse.

For at least a month, I continued to get up and do the same thing. I hadn't even noticed that I was leaving the house in my pajamas with no shoes or socks or even a coat. My housemate made mention of it when she woke up one time when I was about to get into the car. She rode with me to the house, stayed in the car when I got out and looked around, and then we returned home.

It's funny now that I think about it, because she was a police officer, but she was too scared to get out of the car to investigate. Perhaps because I had a spiritual feeling and she didn't.

The significance of those two times will be apparent in the next part of the story.

Fourth Sequence: Mommy's passing

When my mother passed away, it was unexpected. She went into the hospital to have her kidneys checked. This process involved shooting iodine through her system so that the doctors could see the kidney circulation flow.

For reasons I won't get into now, the process did not go as expected. It was an outpatient procedure, but Mommy had to stay in the hospital overnight because she developed a fever. Of course, Daddy was right by her side. She was released the next day, came home and about one and a half days later, she woke up telling Daddy that something didn't feel right.

Daddy took her vitals and decided to take her to the hospital. Mommy had kidney testing procedure done on a Monday. She was back in the hospital on Wednesday. She passed away on Sunday, March 3, 2002, from the complications of an infection.

As sad as we all were that day, there was a rainbow behind the storm. There was good news and reasons to give God all the praise. The good news was that Mommy was able to speak to her children via phone before she passed. I was able to see her that night, had time alone with her so I could pray with her in case her homegoing was near. While she was sleeping or unconscious, not sure which one, as I prayed over her body.

I told her, "I know your body is tired, Mommy, so if you must go, we'll understand. But if you can stay around us for just a little bit to check on us before going to heaven, I really would appreciate it. Like maybe check on everyone. Thanks. And, God, we give our mother to you in the name of Jesus to do your will on earth as it is in heaven."

After saying my prayer, I sat next to her in a chair and watched her sleep. She must have felt the heat of my stare on her face, because she suddenly opened her eyes and saw the worry on my face. She smiled at me and stuck her tongue out. We both laughed.

Being the matriarch of a family of seven, having to take on so much responsibility for our welfare and well-being, Mommy always went out of her way to make sure we were okay. She never wanted us to see her sad. She never wanted us to worry, forever apologizing when she had seizures or maybe a small toileting. Her transition was no different. She didn't want me to worry, so she did something to make me smile. How wonderful of my mother to do that for me. To think of me, right then.

Mommy was also able to talk to Sharon that night over the phone, using all the air she could muster up in her lungs to make her conversation sound normal instead of weak. She was really weak at this time and on oxygen. She smiled while talking to Sharon. Beautiful.

I was able to kiss her goodnight at midnight before leaving the hospital, a kiss I delivered for all my brothers and sister, and her sister and father, who could not be there at that time.

Interestingly, as I was leaving the hospital room, my housemate, who was with me, said, "Okay, Mrs. Collins. We'll see you later."

Mommy responded, "Are you sure about that, girlfriend?"

My housemate replied, "Yes, I'm sure."

"Hmmph," Mommy said, like she knew a secret no one else did. Mommy made other statements before her passing that led me to believe that she, too, knew that peace was coming.

On that night, in the wee hours of the morning before she passed, Daddy held her against his chest and rubbed her back.

Mommy slowly lifted her head to look at Daddy. "I love you."

"I love you too, baby," Daddy responded.

"Now, lay me down, Cliff. I'm tired."

Daddy gently laid her down on the bed, and moments later, she went into cardiac arrest. It was quick. From my understanding, by the time they moved her to the elevator and down just three floors, Mommy had passed.

We are truly grateful that Mommy didn't suffer. We are grateful Daddy was there the entire time, and we were grateful for the life our mother lived. Although we would have loved to have had her with us for another forty years or more, that was not to be. She had lived a very productive and quality life.

Knowing what we learned about the results of the kidney test, Mommy probably wouldn't have lived the life she was accustomed to up until the time of her passing. After the stroke, my parents still had fun, traveled, laughed and did things they had always done. Had Mommy lived, she probably would have endured countless doctor's visits, and the quality of her life would have diminished greatly. Mommy would not have been happy. We never wanted to see that.

Although her passing was unexpected, when I look back on the series of events, I believe there were signs. The strange but loving phone call from Mommy that she said she didn't make. The "dream" that Daddy had that Mommy was calling him. Mommy's response when my housemate said that we would see her later. Even the times that I got up in the middle of the night to search for something at our old house. Well, Mommy had a heart attack at 3:45 a.m. and was pronounced dead at 4:15 a.m.—the same times I kept waking up.

What am I saying? What does this mean? To me, it means that no matter what you do or try to do, like the animals that surround us who have this sixth sense of "knowing" when their time has come, we, too, can feel something.

It also means that you can go ahead and live your life to the fullest. No need to worry about the coming of peace. When it comes, it comes. It is written in the books. So, enjoy life together as much as you can and don't look back!

I see it all as being reconnected to God. To return to where you began. Just like other times when you can tell something you ate didn't sit right with you, or perhaps someone's energy is kind of quirky, but you have never met them before in your life, your body and spirit speak to you in times of crisis and "homegoings."

When Mommy's time came, there was no more suffering, pain or medical challenges of any kind anymore. Her spirit spoke to her, and it spoke to us, her loved ones, and then she was free. As a special bonus, knowing how Mommy passed taught me how I wanted to live and how I wanted to love and be loved. I want to be loved by someone who would never leave me, always be there for me through my trials, struggles and victories and would be there to rub my back, profess their undying love to me, kiss me, then lay me down to sleep. That would be beautiful.

I base my decisions on partnerships based on the lessons of my parents' partnership and enduring love. So again, knowing how Mommy passed taught me how I wanted to live.

Angels Watching Over Us All, The Spirituality of It All

I was truly grateful for all the aforementioned incidents that occurred before my mother passed. Yet, I really had a hard time for a while. I took care of Mommy the best I could, but still, I wondered if I could have done more. Daddy had similar questions rolling around in his head.

For a long time, I wept and grieved every day. I tried to maintain a sense of normalcy. I went to work, but I cried in my office or when I got home. I missed Mommy so. I still had many questions. What went wrong? What could I have done? I cried myself to sleep, replaying everything over and over in my head, hoping that, this time, maybe I would see something that I could have done differently that would have saved her life. I didn't know what I was searching for, exactly. When I think about it now, if I had the answer to what went wrong, it wouldn't bring Mommy back. It may have even made me feel worse. All I can say is that I was searching for something . . . something that made sense to explain something that made no sense to me at all. So, I kept searching and questioning.

I talked to Mommy, in my head and sometimes out loud. I wasn't going to allow death to keep me away from my mother.

Not too long after Mommy passed, I bought my first house. Six bedrooms, two and half bathrooms, den, formal dining room, living room, two-car garage, a huge kitchen and a front and backyard. I grieved, laughed and prayed in every room. Eventually, I was really tired of, well, crying. But I was afraid that if I stopped crying, grieving and honoring Mommy in some way, I would forget about her. I would forget about her birthday or special moments. So, I hung onto the pain.

Not consciously. It wasn't intentional. Looking back, it was almost like I just couldn't let go and wasn't going to let go until I was done or until God or Mommy told me to stop crying and asking questions.

One Final Sequence

After Mommy's passing, I had this dream, or what I would call a vision—an experience really. I was asleep in bed when Mommy came to me in a dream, and she was smiling. When I looked at her with what felt like my third eye, she appeared to be around twenty-five years old or so. Just absolutely beautiful. Flawless. She spoke to me, and I understood what she was saying although she didn't speak with her mouth. It was like we were talking through our thoughts.

The next thing I knew, I was in Mommy's hospital room. I looked to my left, and Mommy was smiling at me from the corner of the room. To the right, I saw her body on the bed, just the way I remember her when she was leaving us. Her eyes were closed, but she was still alive. The whole room was filled with nurses and doctors just walking around or sitting. The room was packed, maybe thirty to thirty-five people. They all had clipboards.

I turned back to my left, and a woman was standing in front of me, slightly to my side. She was a rather tall, attractive, white woman with brown-reddish hair and a pleasant smile. I would call her an Irish beauty. She began to speak, using her mouth.

"Your mother tells us you've been having a hard time letting go. You're concerned you didn't do enough, and you had a lot of questions."

"Yes. That's right," I responded, not scared at all.

I smiled while I listened to her and responded with my mind and my mouth.

She continued. "We are here to help you. What you didn't know was that she had two extra conditions that affected the doctor's ability to help her. All these nurses, doctors and specialists that you see in this room are angels who have passed on and are now here, trying to help your mother. We have kidney specialists, heart specialists and all types of specialists, and they were all called here to try and help your mother."

I looked around at them, watching them work. Not one of them noticed me or looked up from what they were doing. Some were standing up. Some were pacing, and some were sitting on the sides and at end of Mommy's bed.

The Irish beauty went on. "When someone goes through an ordeal like this, angels come in to see if they can fix things. They try everything. If they have done all they can and can't find a cure, or if they can't help the situation, then a decision is made as to whether the person's quality of life would be better here on earth or in heaven. If their quality of life would suffer here and we have done everything that we can do, then they are called home."

She spoke with such knowledge and authority, hearing what she was telling me felt reassuring, kind and soft. I was thinking that maybe she was the senior doctor on this trip.

"Your mother had two conditions. They were _____ and _____. We worked to fix the problem to save your mother." (I have to leave blanks when it comes to the medical terms she told me, because the words were so long. I had never heard of these conditions before, nor have I ever seen the words before that moment. I still can't remember what they were.)

"Unless your doctors knew of these two conditions, they really couldn't help her. It was missed and kind of rare. But we don't give up until we have tried everything. Everyone here is the best in their specific fields, and as you can see, they are trying their best to save your mother."

I turned to look at Mommy's spirit still smiling on the left side of the room.

I suddenly began to understand. Mommy smiled at me as the doctor said, "We had to bring your mother home. It was for the best. You did everything that could have been done. You, your father, sister, everyone who tried to help. It was just her time. That's all. Do you understand now?"

"Yes, I do," I replied.

"Do you feel better now?"

"Yes, thank you very much."

"Good," she said warmly.

I then turned to Mommy who was still smiling at me. This time, her smile glowed like there was peace now, from her to me, and now, within me. I smiled at her and telepathically said, "Thank you, Mommy."

Her bright, warm and loving smile said, "You're welcome," and it was over.

I woke up. Because I have photogenic memory, I quickly wrote down the two words that the doctor showed me on her clipboard as quickly as I could so I wouldn't forget them. They were twelve letters long and sixteen letters long. I didn't know if I was dreaming or if what happened was real. A real vision and conversation.

Sweating a little, I went to my computer and typed in the first word that I had never seen before in my life. I waited for the search engine to do its thing and . . . *voila!* There it was! The first word and exactly how she explained the meaning and condition. I typed in the second word. It happened again. I couldn't believe it! How is this even possible? But it had to be real. I had to believe what I experienced, because there was no other way to explain what just happened with such precision, detail and full information.

I become overwhelmed with joy! More joy than Mr. Scrooge could have ever felt knowing of Christmas past. Mommy made it! Mommy made it! She made it to heaven and is in pristine condition—young, vibrant and alive! I was really happy! From that moment, I didn't feel anymore guilt or depression like I had before. I never cried in that same grieving and mourning way again. In fact, I felt I had been healed. The blessing continued.

One day, when Daddy was feeling down, questioning if he did enough, I was able to look him straight in his eyes and tell him, "Daddy, there was nothing you could do. It was just Mommy's time. You did everything you could humanly do. Now, she's in heaven, a traveling spirit, helping someone get through something."

I told him a little about my vision so he would understand why I was so confident about what I was saying. I didn't say too much, because I didn't want him to feel uncomfortable about hearing spiritual things like this. His feelings were still raw. So, I told him just enough to console him in some way that Mommy was indeed okay.

It truly was and is a blessing to know there are angels watching over us, and I love it. The spirituality of it all.

What did I learn? Know that you are never alone. There are always angels around you, helping you in everyday life and when you are in a time of need. Rest assured, they are sending some of the best to your rescue, filling up your room with love and support, working for your good. It's okay.

One extra gem for you as a sidenote. Remember that six-bedroom house that I bought? People were always asking or making comments about why I, as a single woman, needed all that house, all those rooms. I sold it.

After a year of praying and healing in every single room over my mother's passing, I decided to go back to school in Ohio to earn my master's degree and doctorate. I sold it on the first day to a family of a Navy man who was being shipped off to sea. He wanted to buy a house in a safe neighborhood for his family before he left. It just so happened that they had also taken into their home, a woman and her children who had been going through some difficulties in her marriage.

I sold the house to the family that very night; they needed exactly six bedrooms. That's why I needed that house. To help prepare it for those families.

Riding the Rainbow

There are no mistakes in the work and blessings of God. All was well. All is well.

Thank you, Mommy. Thank you, God Jehovah, and thank you to the angels from above, Heaven-sent, to watch over us.

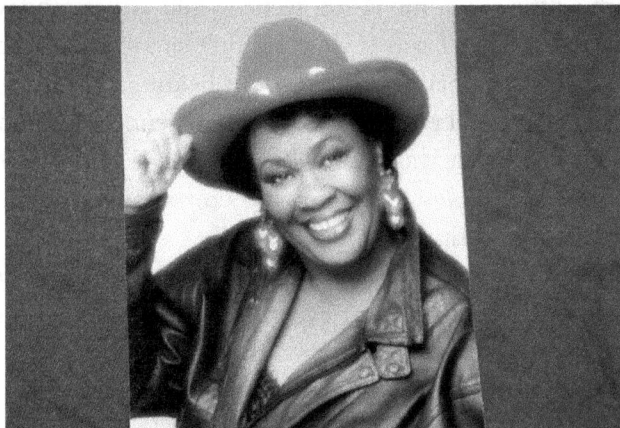

Viola Collins (April 28, 1937 - March 3, 2002)

About the Author

Dr. Janice Collins is a Kopenhaver Fellow and earned a Ph.D. in Communications from the Scripps College of Communications at Ohio University, specializing in Media Management and Critical Cultural Theory with an Associate Certification in Women's Studies. She earned a Master's of Science and Women's Studies Certification at the E.W. Scripps School of Journalism at Ohio University and a Bachelor of Arts degree in Speech Communications and Theatre Arts with a concentration in Communication/Rhetoric and a certification in Women's Studies at Wake Forest University.

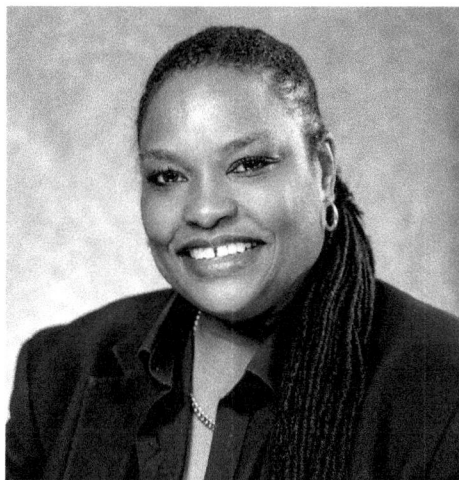

A human conglomerate, Dr. Collins has won multi-national and international awards as a journalist, documentarian, producer, director, writer, editor, cinematographer, reporter, professor, scholar, researcher of mixed methodology and creative. She works as a media and leadership practitioner, expert and consultant, and enjoys empowering others as a motivational speaker and a pedagogy expert on diversity, equity, belonging, and inclusion (DEBI).

She founded and created Active Centralized Empowerment (A.C.E.), a national, award-winning, critical pedagogy and organizational design for inclusion and equity that she developed over eighteen years. A.C.E. is one of the only DEBI initiatives designed for full and holistic inclusion of all participants.

Her book, *Teaching without Borders,* is written for the educator who believes that each student carries value and something special to offer to the world. Her cooking podcast, Seasoned with Love, was named after the informal catering service she and her mother started during her mother's recovery.

Dr. Collins was recently selected as one of Gaia International Alliance Humanity Leader Top Picks. Gaia International Alliance is a Foundation created to recognize top leaders and experts in the field of humanity, transformation, spirituality and all aspects of the healing arts.

As a military brat from a huge Christian family of eight, she has always believed that each person is born with a special gift, something only they can give to the world. One of her gifts is the ability to see a person's heart. She loves to love others and see people reach their highest potential, fulfillment and happiness.

Connect with Janice Collins at:
drcollins@wcmif.org
aceactivated@outlook.com
drcollins@teaching-without-borders.org